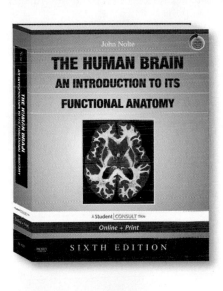
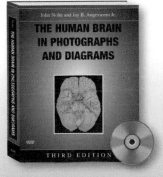
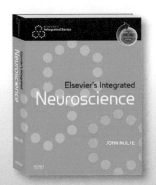

Essentials
of the
Human Brain

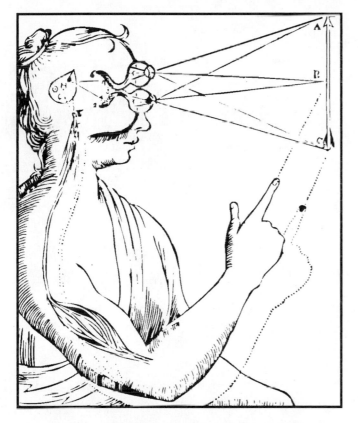

Reproduction of a drawing by Rene Descartes in **De Homine**, 1662. Descartes thought that the pineal gland was the seat of the soul, monitoring the movement of "animal spirits" in sensory nerves and controlling the movement of animal spirits through motor nerves.

Essentials of the Human Brain

John Nolte, PhD

Professor of Cell Biology and Anatomy
The University of Arizona College of Medicine
Tucson, Arizona

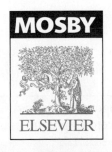

MOSBY

ELSEVIER

1600 John F. Kennedy Blvd.
Ste 1800
Philadelphia, PA 19103-2899

ESSENTIALS OF THE HUMAN BRAIN   ISBN 978-0-323-04570-4

Notice

Neither the Publisher nor the Editor assumes any responsibility for any loss or injury and/or damage to persons or property arising out of or related to any use of the material contained in this book. It is the responsibility of the treating practitioner, relying on independent expertise and knowledge of the patient, to determine the best treatment and method of application for the patient.

The Publisher

Library of Congress Cataloging-in-Publication Data

Nolte, John.
   Essentials of the human brain / John Nolte.
      p. ; cm.
   ISBN 978-0-323-04570-4
   1. Brain.   2. Neuroanatomy.   I. Title.
   [DNLM: 1. Nervous System—anatomy & histology.   2. Brain—physiology.   3. Nervous
System Physiology. WL 101 N798e 2010]
   QP376.N655 2010
   612.8′2—dc22

                                                      2008049005

Acquisitions Editor: Madelene Hyde
Developmental Editor: Andrew Hall
Publishing Services Manager: Linda Van Pelt
Design Direction: Gene Harris

Printed in Canada

Last digit is the print number: 9 8 7 6 5 4 3 2 1

Preface

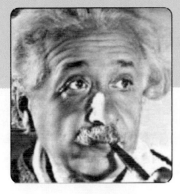

Everything should be made as simple as possible, but not simpler.
Albert Einstein

This is a book for students. Specifically, it is a book for students trying to review neuroscience or to distill out the important facts and concepts of human neuroscience. I tried to make it an account that would be useful by itself, so it does not depend too much on *The Human Brain* (Elsevier/Mosby, sixth edition, 2009) to make sense. However, it does parallel *The Human Brain* in its organization and should be particularly useful when used in conjunction with that book. Each chapter begins with an outline and includes key concepts boxes distributed through the text; collectively these are very similar to the outline at the beginning of the comparable chapter in *The Human Brain*, although some fine points were omitted. In order to keep *Essentials* brief, some background material was left out, so it may not be productive to read the book with no prior knowledge of the subject. At the end of each chapter is a list of a few questions dealing specifically with the content of that chapter. Toward the end of the book, Appendix 1 is a longer list of questions that often cover multiple topics. Whenever the answer to a question is not a simple definition or fact, a brief explanation is included in Appendix 2. The clinical questions are fictions that are meant to illustrate neurobiological concepts. They are not intended to be clinically accurate or to make light of neurological disease. There are references here and there to figures in this *Essentials* book and also to figures in the sixth edition of *The Human Brain*. In order to differentiate between them, figures in *The Human Brain* are set off in magenta and are referred to as "THB6 Figure__," and *Essentials* figures are referred to as "Fig.__." I also added a section of blank drawings at the very end of the book as Appendix 3; you may find these useful for drawing out pathways and connections.

I wanted to call this book *Translucent Neuroscience* (the publisher wouldn't let me), in the hope that it makes a difficult subject almost clear. What I tried to do is list and explain succinctly the really crucial material in *The Human Brain*. I did it mainly by compiling and adapting the list of learning objectives dealing with neurobiological topics that we use in the course I teach at The University of Arizona College of Medicine. My list is unlikely to coincide exactly with that used by others, but it should overlap substantially.

My hope is that the chapter outlines and key concepts define the core material clearly, the text explains this material lucidly, and the questions at the end of each chapter and the explanations near the end of the book will allow you to determine your level of understanding with some confidence. I welcome comments on content or format, from students or faculty, so that the next version can be nearly transparent.

As always, I owe thanks to many people for their help. Students who have taken my courses in years past have helped hone and clarify the content. Past and present teaching colleagues, especially Jay Angevine, Ray Carmody, Pam Eller, Tom Finger, Kati Gothard, Gail Koshland, Erwin Montgomery, Jeremy Payne, Frank Porreca, Steve Ringel, Scott Sherman, Todd Vanderah, and Steve Wright, provided insights that had evaded me. Elsevier was kind enough to let me borrow or simplify many figures from *The Human Brain* for use in this book. Harry and the rest of the handball players provided mental therapy. Kathy makes me happy every day.

John Nolte
Tucson, Arizona, August 2008

Contents

Introduction to the Nervous System

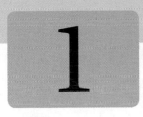

The brain seems bewilderingly complex the first few times you look at it. One way to ease the bewilderment is to have an overview of some vocabulary and organizing principles, which the first three chapters of this book attempt to provide. Chapter 1 is a quick introduction to the parts of the nervous system and the cells that make it up, Chapter 2 is an overview of how the parts get arranged that way during development, and Chapter 3 is a closer look at major parts and the wiring principles underlying their interconnections.

The Nervous System Has Central and Peripheral Parts

The nervous system has both central and peripheral parts, roughly corresponding to the parts inside and outside the skull and vertebral column. The **peripheral nervous system** (**PNS**) is approximately the same thing as the collection of nerves that reach pretty much every part of the head and body, collecting sensory information and delivering messages to body parts or to PNS neurons. The **central nervous system** (**CNS**) is made up of the **brain** and the **spinal cord**. The brain in turn is composed of the **cerebrum (forebrain)**, **cerebellum**, and **brainstem** (Fig. 1-1, Table 1-1). The cerebrum, by far the largest component, is itself composed of two **cerebral hemispheres** and the **diencephalon** (from a Greek word meaning "in-between-brain," because it's interposed between the cerebral hemispheres and the brainstem).

Each cerebral hemisphere has a covering of **cerebral cortex** and encloses a series of large nuclei. Some of the enclosed nuclei (**lenticular** and **caudate nuclei**) are parts of the **basal ganglia**, which help control movement; another (the **amygdala**) is part of the **limbic system**, which deals with drives and emotions. The cerebral cortex is a critical structure for perception, for the initiation of voluntary movement, and for the functions we think of as distinctively human—things like language and reasoning. Corresponding to these several

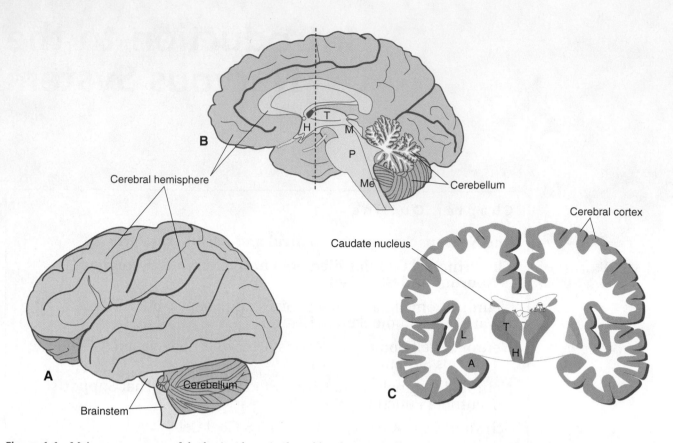

Figure 1-1   Major components of the brain (the spinal cord has been cut off at its junction with the brainstem). **A,** The left side of a brain; anterior is to the left. **B,** The right half of a hemisected brain; anterior is to the left. **C,** A coronal section of a cerebrum, in the plane indicated in B. *A,* Amygdala; *H,* hypothalamus; *L,* lenticular nucleus; *M,* midbrain; *Me,* medulla; *P,* pons; *T,* thalamus.

Table 1-1	Major divisions of the brain	
Major Division	**Subdivision**	**Principal Function**
Cerebral hemisphere	Cerebral cortex	Perception, cognition, memory, voluntary movement
	Lenticular nucleus	Part of the basal ganglia: movement control
	Caudate nucleus	Part of the basal ganglia: movement control
	Amygdala	Part of the limbic system: drives and emotions
Diencephalon	Thalamus	Relays information to the cerebral cortex
	Hypothalamus	Controls the autonomic nervous system
Brainstem	Midbrain	Cranial nerve nuclei, long tracts
	Pons	Cranial nerve nuclei, long tracts
	Medulla	Cranial nerve nuclei, long tracts
Cerebellum		Coordination of movement

functions, there are cortical areas primarily concerned with sensation, others with movement, and still others with more complex activities. Because of this parceling of functions, it is possible for cortical damage to impair some abilities while leaving others more or less unaffected.

The diencephalon includes the **thalamus**, a relay station for information on its way to the cerebral cortex, and the **hypothalamus**, which controls the **autonomic nervous system** and many aspects of drive-related behavior. The brainstem is subdivided into the **midbrain**, **pons**, and **medulla**. It contains most of the **cranial nerve nuclei**, as well as **long tracts** on their way to or from the cerebrum. The cerebellum is interconnected with many other parts of the CNS and, like the basal ganglia, helps control movement.

Table 1-2	Major cell types of the nervous system	
Location	**Major Neurons**	**Major Glia**

CNS	Motor neurons (→ skeletal muscle via PNS)
	 Preganglionic autonomic neurons (→ autonomic
	  ganglia via PNS)
	 Interneurons
	  local interneurons
	  projection neurons
		Astrocytes (metabolic support, response to injury)
		 Oligodendrocytes (myelin)
		 Ependymal cells (line ventricles, secrete CSF)
		 Microglia (response to injury)

PNS	Primary sensory neurons (spinal, cranial nerve, and enteric
	  ganglia)
	 Postganglionic autonomic neurons (sympathetic,
	  parasympathetic, and enteric ganglia)
		Schwann cells (myelin, satellite cells)

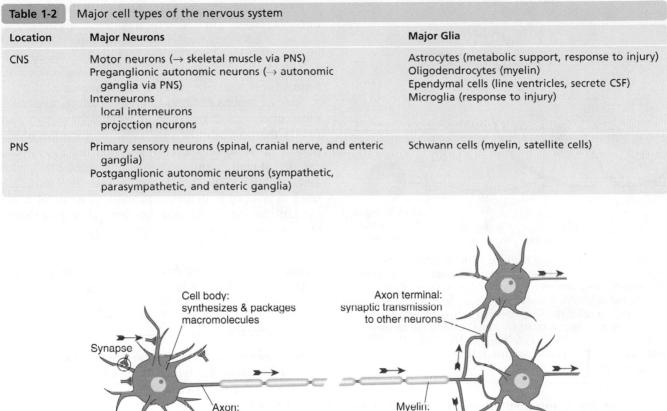

Cell body: synthesizes & packages macromolecules

Axon terminal: synaptic transmission to other neurons

Synapse

Axon: conducts action potentials toward other neurons

Myelin: glial covering that speeds conduction

Dendrites: site of most (but not all) synaptic inputs

Figure 1-2 Principal components of a typical neuron.

The Principal Cellular Elements of the Nervous System Are Neurons and Glial Cells

Except for some extrinsic elements such as blood and blood vessels (see Chapter 6) and meninges (see Chapter 4), the whole nervous system is made up of just two general categories of cells: **neurons** and **glial cells** (or **glia**). Each can be divided into a few subcategories, some characteristic of the CNS and others of the PNS (Table 1-2; see THB6 Fig. 1-27, p. 27).

Neurons Come in a Variety of Sizes and Shapes, but All Are Variations on the Same Theme

Although there are lots of variations, a typical neuron (Fig. 1-2) has a collection of tapering **dendrites** and a single cylindrical **axon**, all emerging from the **cell body**. The cell body is the synthetic center of the whole neuron, the dendrites receive most of the inputs

(**synapses**) from other neurons, the axon conducts electrical impulses (**action potentials**) away from the cell body and toward other neurons, and **axon terminals** release **neurotransmitter** onto other neurons. So the anatomical polarization (dendrites → cell body → axon) corresponds to a functional polarization in terms of the direction in which electrical signals move.

Nearly all neurons fall into one of six categories (Fig. 1-3):

1. **Sensory neurons**, such as those in dorsal root and cranial nerve ganglia, deliver information to the CNS. The cell bodies live in the PNS, but processes extend through both the PNS and CNS.
2. **Motor neurons** have cell bodies in the CNS and axons that travel through the PNS to reach skeletal muscle.
3. **Preganglionic autonomic neurons** have cell bodies in the CNS and axons that travel through the PNS to reach autonomic ganglia.

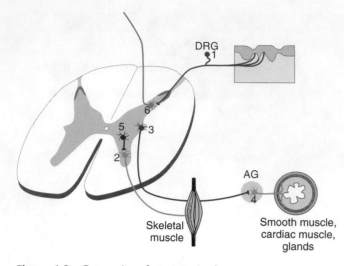

Figure 1-3 Categories of neurons in the nervous system, as seen in the spinal cord. Some neurons do not fit comfortably into one of these categories (e.g., rods and cones of the retina), but most do. *1*, Sensory neurons, in this case a dorsal root ganglion cell (DRG); *2*, motor neurons; *3*, preganglionic autonomic neurons; *4*, postganglionic autonomic neurons, with cell bodies in autonomic ganglia (AG); *5*, local interneurons; *6*, projection neurons.

4. **Postganglionic autonomic neurons** have cell bodies in the PNS (in autonomic ganglia) and axons that travel through the PNS to reach smooth muscle, cardiac muscle, and glands.
5. **Local interneurons** are entirely contained in the CNS and have short axons that project to nearby CNS areas.
6. **Projection neurons** are also contained entirely within the CNS, but they have long axons that project in bundles to distant CNS areas.

It's a little arbitrary deciding how long an axon has to be before it qualifies as belonging to a projection neuron, but between them local interneurons and projection neurons account for more than 99% of all our neurons.

Neuronal Cell Bodies and Axons Are Largely Segregated Within the Nervous System

The CNS is mostly separated into areas of **gray matter**, containing neuronal cell bodies and dendrites, and areas of **white matter**, containing axons. Most synapses are made onto neuronal dendrites and cell bodies, so gray matter contains the sites of neural information processing and white matter is like telephone cables interconnecting these sites.

A specific area of gray matter is most often referred to as a **nucleus** (e.g., the trigeminal motor nucleus contains motor neurons for jaw muscles); when it forms a surface covering, it may be referred to as a **cortex** (e.g., cerebral cortex, cerebellar cortex). **Ganglion** ("swelling") usually

refers to a group of neuronal cell bodies in the peripheral nervous system, but is also used occasionally to refer to masses of CNS gray matter (e.g., basal ganglia). There is also an assortment of other names based on the appearance or location of an area of gray matter (e.g., thalamus, from a Greek word meaning "inner chamber").

Specific groups of fibers in areas of white matter are most often called **tracts**, and usually have two-part names that indicate the origin and termination of the fibers. For example, the corticospinal tract consists of axons that emerge from neurons in the cerebral cortex and terminate in the spinal cord. Several other terms are used to refer to structurally prominent areas of white matter; the most common are **fasciculus**, **lemniscus**, and **peduncle**.

Neuronal Organelles Are Distributed in a Pattern That Supports Neuronal Function

> **Key Concepts**
>
> Neuronal cell bodies synthesize macromolecules.
> Dendrites receive synaptic inputs.
> Axons convey electrical signals over long distances.
> Organelles and macromolecules are transported in both directions along axons.
> Synaptic contacts mediate information transfer between neurons.

Neurons deal with the same issues as other cells, using the same organelles (Fig. 1-4). However, some of these issues are accentuated because of the specialized structure and function of neurons:

1. Neurons are electrical signaling machines (see Chapters 7 and 8), so they need to control ionic concentration gradients, pumping in the opposite direction ions that enter or leave as part of an electrical signaling process or just leak across the membrane. This requires a lot of energy and a lot of mitochondria.
2. Many neurons are huge in the longitudinal dimension because of their long axons and extensive dendrites, but they have only one cell body and one nucleus. So the cell body is constantly busy synthesizing enzymes, other proteins, and organelles for the rest of the neuron; this too requires a lot of energy and a lot of mitochondria, as well as a lot of endoplasmic reticulum and ribosomes (appearing as **Nissl bodies**). Diffusion of things like proteins and organelles along an axon would be much too slow, so there are active mechanisms for transporting them. Soluble substances move a few mm/day

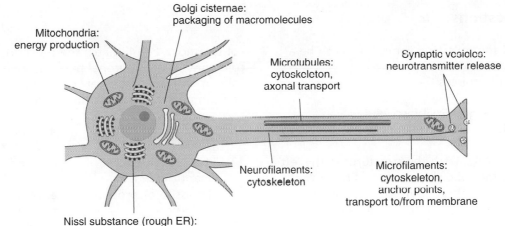

Figure 1-4 Major organelles of a typical neuron.

by **slow axonal transport**. Membrane-associated components move by **fast axonal transport** (about a hundred times faster), using **microtubules** as "railroad tracks."

3. Neurons, like other cells, are largely bags of water encased by a microscopically thin membrane, so maintaining their elaborate shapes is a trick. To do this, they construct a cytoskeleton from filamentous proteins—microtubules, **neurofilaments** (neuronal intermediate filaments), and **microfilaments** (actin).

4. Neurons convey electrical signals to other neurons by dumping small quantities of chemicals (neurotransmitters) onto them. This requires a specialized, very fast secretory process at synapses.

Schwann Cells Are the Principal PNS Glial Cells

> ### Key Concept
>
> PNS axons can be myelinated or unmyelinated.

Schwann cells envelop PNS neurons and their axons in three different ways. Some Schwann cells are flattened out as **satellite cells** that surround PNS ganglion cells (THB6 Figure 1-22, p. 23). Others have multiple indentations, each encasing part of a small (**unmyelinated**) axon (THB6 Figure 1-26, p. 26). Finally, many spiral around individual, larger axons (THB6 Figures 1-23 to 1-25, pp. 24 and 25), forming **myelin sheaths** that allow axons to conduct action potentials more rapidly (see Chapter 7). Each myelinated axon looks like a string of sausages, each sausage being a length of axon covered by the myelin formed by a single Schwann cell; the constrictions between sausages correspond to **nodes of Ranvier**, gaps in the myelin where nerve impulses are regenerated.

CNS Glial Cells Include Oligodendrocytes, Astrocytes, Ependymal Cells, and Microglial Cells

> ### Key Concepts
>
> Some CNS axons are myelinated by oligodendrocytes, but others are unmyelinated.
> Astrocytes provide structural and metabolic support to neurons.
> Ependymal cells line the ventricles.
> Microglial cells respond to CNS injury.

Oligodendrocytes form myelin sheaths in the CNS. In contrast to Schwann cells, individual oligodendrocytes have multiple branches, each ending as a segment of myelin around a different axon (THB6 Figures 1-30 and 1-31, pp. 29 and 30).

Astrocytes play multiple roles, generally less well understood than that of oligodendrocytes. Their cytoskeletons provide mechanical support to neighboring neurons. Astrocyte processes cover the parts of neurons not occupied by synaptic contacts and help regulate the ionic composition of extracellular fluids. They also contact CNS capillaries and help regulate local blood flow (see Chapter 6), and they assist in neuronal metabolism in multiple ways. Finally, they hypertrophy in response to CNS injury and form a kind of scar tissue (see Chapter 24).

Ependymal cells form the single-cell-thick lining of the **ventricles** (the fluid-filled cavities inside the CNS; see Chapter 5). At some locations they are specialized as a secretory epithelium that produces the **cerebrospinal fluid** that fills the ventricles.

Microglia form a sort of immune system within the CNS. They recognize damaged neural tissue and foreign invaders, proliferate, and clean things up.

Study Questions

1. Which of the following is most likely to be a gray matter structure?
   a. Lateral lemniscus
   b. Putamen
   c. Medial longitudinal fasciculus
   d. Superior cerebellar peduncle

For questions 2-5, match the structures in the left column with the subdivisions of the CNS in the column on the right; a subdivision can be used once, more than once, or not at all.

2. Lenticular nucleus   a. Cerebral hemisphere
3. Pons   b. Diencephalon
4. Hypothalamus   c. Brainstem
5. Amygdala   d. Cerebellum

For questions 6-10, match the functions or structures in the left column with the cell types in the column on the right; a cell type can be used once, more than once, or not at all.

6. CNS myelin sheaths   a. Astrocytes
7. PNS myelin sheaths   b. Ependymal cells
8. Phagocytosis of infectious organisms   c. Microglia
   d. Neurons
9. Secretion of cerebrospinal fluid   e. Oligodendrocytes
   f. Schwann cells
10. Glial covering of unmyelinated PNS axons

For questions 11-14, match the functions in the left column with the neuronal parts or organelles in the column on the right; a part or organelle can be used once, more than once, or not at all.

11. Substrate for fast axonal transport   a. Axon
   b. Axon terminals
12. Sites receiving most synaptic contacts   c. Dendrites
   d. Microfilaments
13. Major site of protein synthesis   e. Microtubules
   f. Neurofilaments
14. Major sites of neurotransmitter release   g. Nissl bodies

Development of the Nervous System

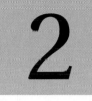

Understanding a little bit about the embryology of the brain helps clarify the way it's put together in adults. The CNS starts out as a simple ectodermal tube that develops some folds and bulges. The cavity of the tube persists as the ventricles, and the folds and bulges determine the shape and layout of many parts of the CNS.

The Neural Tube and Neural Crest Give Rise to the Central and Peripheral Nervous Systems

Cells of the **neural crest** grow at the apex of each **neural fold**. When the neural folds fuse to form the **neural tube**, the neural crest becomes a detached layer between the neural tube and the surface ectoderm (Fig. 2-1). Neural crest cells migrate from there, and go on to form most

neurons and glial cells of the PNS (and much more). These include the sensory neurons of spinal and most cranial nerve ganglia, postganglionic autonomic neurons, and the Schwann cells of peripheral nerves and ganglia (Fig. 2-2). The neural tube goes on to form the CNS.

The Sulcus Limitans Separates Sensory and Motor Areas of the Spinal Cord and Brainstem

The **sulcus limitans** is a longitudinal groove that develops in the lateral wall of the embryonic spinal cord and extends into the **rhombencephalon** (the embryonic medulla and pons, as discussed a little later). It separates two groups of neuronal cell bodies, the **alar plate** (dorsal to the sulcus limitans in the spinal cord) and the **basal plate** (ventral to the sulcus limitans in the spinal cord). The alar and basal plates go on to become sensory and

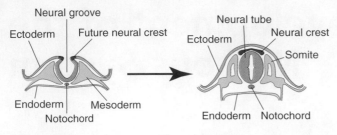

Figure 2-1 Neural groove and neural tube.

motor structures, respectively (Fig. 2-3). The spinal alar plate becomes the **posterior horn**, where primary sensory neurons terminate. The spinal basal plate becomes the **anterior horn**, where the cell bodies of motor neurons live.

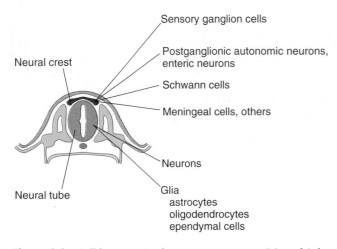

Figure 2-2 Cell lineages in the nervous system. (Most think that microglia are derived from monocyte-related stem cells rather than the neural tube, but this is not known for sure.)

The walls of the neural tube are spread apart in the rhombencephalon, forming the floor of the **fourth ventricle**, so in the medulla and pons the alar plate ends up *lateral* to the basal plate (Fig. 2-4). The same development into sensory and motor structures occurs, however, so cranial nerve sensory nuclei are lateral to cranial nerve motor nuclei in the adult brainstem (see Fig. 12-2).

The Neural Tube Has a Series of Bulges and Flexures

Key Concepts

There are three primary vesicles.
There are five secondary vesicles.
The cavity of the neural tube persists as a system of ventricles.

As the neural tube closes, it develops a series of three bulges called **primary vesicles**. The walls of these three vesicles go on to form the entire brain, and their continuous cavity forms the ventricular system. Because in many ways the CNS retains much of the longitudinal organization of the neural tube, these vesicles provide some useful functional terminology for different CNS regions. The most rostral primary vesicle is the **prosencephalon** (Greek for "front-brain" or **forebrain**), followed by the **mesencephalon** or **midbrain**, followed by the **rhombencephalon** or **hindbrain**, which merges with the embryonic spinal cord. The rhombencephalon is named for the rhomboid fourth ventricle that it contains.

The prosencephalon and rhombencephalon each divides into two **secondary vesicles**, so there is a total of five secondary vesicles. The prosencephalon forms the **telencephalon** ("end-brain") and the **diencephalon**

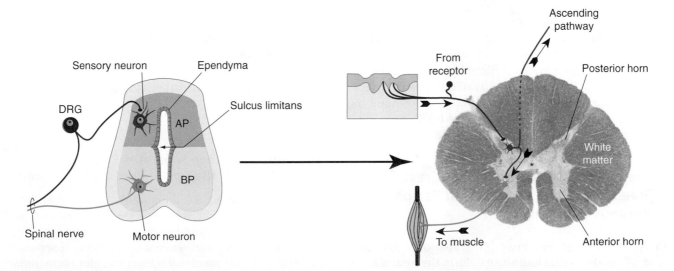

Figure 2-3 Development of the alar (AP) and basal (BP) plates of the embryonic spinal cord into sensory and motor regions of the mature spinal cord. *Central canal of the spinal cord (the remnant of the cavity of the neural tube, where the sulcus limitans used to be); *DRG,* dorsal root ganglion cell.

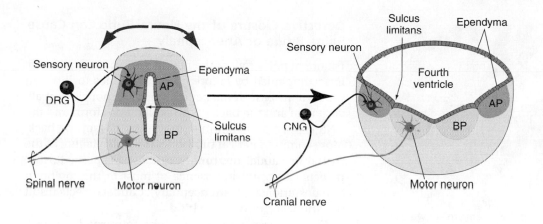

Figure 2-4 Spreading apart of the walls of the neural tube in the medulla and pons results in the alar (AP) and basal (BP) plates winding up in the floor of the fourth ventricle. *CNG*, Cranial nerve ganglion cell; *DRG*, dorsal root ganglion cell.

("in-between-brain"). The telencephalon gives rise to the two cerebral hemispheres, whose cavities become the **lateral ventricles**. The diencephalon gives rise to the thalamus, hypothalamus, **retina**, pineal gland, and several other structures; its cavity becomes the **third ventricle**. The mesencephalon remains undivided as the midbrain; its cavity persists as the **cerebral aqueduct**, which interconnects the third and fourth ventricles. The rhombencephalon forms the **metencephalon** and the **myelencephalon**, which together give rise to the cerebellum and the rest of the brainstem, and enclose the fourth ventricle. This ventricular arrangement is shown schematically in Fig. 2-5 and more realistically in THB6 Figures 5-1 and 5-2, pp. 100 and 101.

Bends in the neural tube also determine some aspects of the shape of the adult brain. Two bends are particularly important: the **pontine flexure** causes the walls of the neural tube to separate and form the floor of the fourth ventricle (see Fig. 2-4), and the **cephalic flexure** persists as the bend between the long axes of the prosencephalon (cerebrum) and the rest of the CNS (see Fig. 3-1).

Growth of the Telencephalon Overshadows Other Parts of the Nervous System

The telencephalon grows much more rapidly than the other vesicles. It folds down beside the diencephalon and fuses with it, and some cerebral cortex (the **insula**) develops over the site of fusion (Fig. 2-6). Subsequent growth of the cerebral hemisphere pivots about the insula, and the hemisphere grows around in a C-shaped arc through the parietal, occipital, and temporal lobes. This C shape is more than an anatomical curiosity that

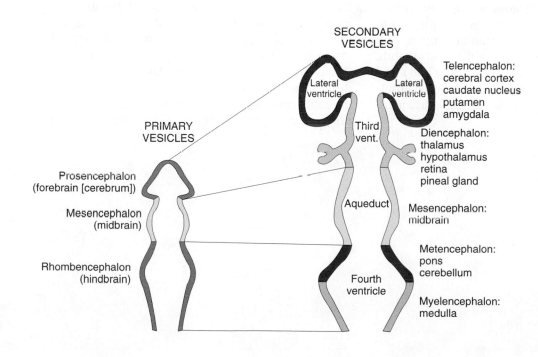

Figure 2-5 Vesicles of the neural tube and some of their major derivatives. The view is if the neural tube had been straightened out and sectioned longitudinally.

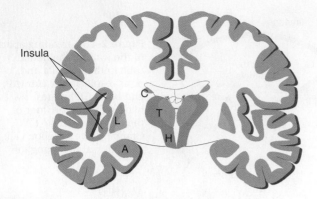

Insula

Figure 2-6   A coronal section of the cerebrum showing the location of the insula, an area of cerebral cortex fused with parts of the basal ganglia and diencephalon and covered over by other cortical areas. *A*, Amygdala; *C*, caudate nucleus; *H*, hypothalamus; *L*, lenticular nucleus; *T*, thalamus.

explains the shape of the lateral ventricles: in some cases, neural structures retain connections to distant sites in the forebrain, and C-shaped tracts interconnecting them are the result (THB6 Figure 3-18, p. 68).

Adverse Events during Development Can Cause Congenital Malformations of the Nervous System

A remarkable array of events has to happen at just the right time in just the right sequence for the CNS to form properly. If something goes wrong, the consequences are related in a reasonably systematic way to the particular stage of the process that's disrupted: formation of the neural tube during the first month, establishment of the basic shape of the brain and facial features during the second month, and massive proliferation and migration of neurons during subsequent months.

Defective Closure of the Neural Tube Can Cause Spina Bifida or Anencephaly

Failure of part or all of the neural tube to close properly is accompanied by failure of nearby bones to form. In the extreme case, if the neural tube does not close at all, vertebrae and the back of the skull do not form and the CNS is open and continuous with the skin of the back. More common **neural tube defects** involve failure of the rostral or caudal **neuropore** to close properly. Rostral defects can result in absence of most of the forebrain and posterior skull (**anencephaly**). Caudal defects result in various forms of **spina bifida**.

Open neural tubes allow **alpha-fetoprotein** to leak out, and increased levels can be detected in amniotic fluid or maternal serum. **Folate** supplements at the time of neural tube closure reduce the incidence of these defects.

Defective Secondary Neurulation Can Cause a Distinctive Set of Abnormalities

The sacral spinal cord forms just after the neural tube closes, by a mechanism involving extension of the cavity of the tube a little farther caudally. Problems with this process can cause a spectrum of abnormalities involving function of the sacral cord; these are typically accompanied by signs in the overlying skin, but not an open neural tube.

The Prosencephalon Can Develop Abnormally Even if Neural Tube Closure Is Complete

Once the neural tube has closed the cerebral hemispheres begin to enlarge, in a process coordinated with facial development. Just as neural tube defects are accompanied by abnormalities of nearby bone, defective development of the telencephalic vesicles into separate cerebral hemispheres is typically accompanied by facial abnormalities. Problems later in development, during the period of proliferation and migration of neurons, may result in profound mental deficits but normal development of the face, skull, and vertebrae.

Study Questions

1. A stillborn infant was noted to have a grossly abnormal skull and cerebrum. The parietal bones, most of the occipital bones, and most of the frontal bones above the orbits were absent; a malformed remnant of the cerebrum, with few recognizable neural structures, was exposed at the site of the skull defect. The most likely cause of this malformation was defective
   a. formation or migration of neural crest cells.
   b. closure of the rostral neuropore.
   c. closure of the caudal neuropore.
   d. separation of the telencephalic vesicles.
   e. proliferation or migration of CNS neurons.

2. A 7-day-old infant was evaluated because of intermittent vomiting that began a day after birth. A barium enema study at 7 days demonstrated contraction of several centimeters of colon near the rectum; a length of colon proximal to the contraction was abnormally distended. Biopsy of the contracted colon wall revealed absence of autonomic ganglion cells. The most likely cause of this disorder was defective
   a. formation or migration of neural crest cells.
   b. closure of the rostral neuropore.
   c. closure of the caudal neuropore.
   d. separation of the telencephalic vesicles.
   e. proliferation or migration of CNS neurons.

3. A 3-month-old with a generally normal face, skull, and head size was evaluated for seizures and developmental delay. An imaging study of the CNS revealed that the basic components of the cerebral hemispheres and diencephalon were present, and the lateral and third ventricles could be visualized easily. However, the cerebral surface was smooth, with an indentation at the site of the insula bilaterally but few or no other sulci or gyri; the lateral ventricles were somewhat enlarged. The most likely cause of this malformation was defective
   a. formation or migration of neural crest cells.
   b. closure of the rostral neuropore.
   c. closure of the caudal neuropore.
   d. separation of the telencephalic vesicles.
   e. proliferation or migration of CNS neurons.

4. Neural crest cells
   a. develop in the roof of the ventricles.
   b. pinch off from the neural folds as the neural tube forms.
   c. pinch off from an outgrowth of the diencephalon.
   d. form the rostral end of the neural tube.

5. Derivatives of the neural crest include
   a. most motor neurons.
   b. the glial cells that form the myelin sheaths of CNS axons.
   c. the primary sensory neurons whose axons travel in spinal nerves.
   d. the cerebral cortex.

For questions 6-10, match the structures in the left column with the neural tube vesicles in the column on the right; choices can be used once, more than once, or not at all.

6. Cerebellum	a. Diencephalon
7. Thalamus	b. Mesencephalon
8. Caudate nucleus	c. Metencephalon
9. Midbrain	d. Myelencephalon
10. Retina	e. Telencephalon

Gross Anatomy and General Organization of the Central Nervous System

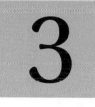

A useful way to start studying the brain is to learn some of the vocabulary that refers to its major parts, and to understand in a vague way what they do. These major parts can then serve as reference points to build on in later chapters.

The Long Axis of the CNS Bends at the Cephalic Flexure

Most creatures move through the world with their spinal cords oriented horizontally. In humans, the cephalic flexure of the embryonic neural tube persists in the adult brain as a bend of about 80° between the midbrain and the diencephalon, allowing us to walk around upright. Terms like **dorsal** and **ventral**, however, are used as though the flexure does not exist, the CNS is still a straight tube, and we walk around on all fours. The result is that in the spinal cord and brainstem dorsal has the same meaning as posterior, whereas in the forebrain dorsal has the same meaning as superior (Fig. 3-1).

Hemisecting a Brain Reveals Parts of the Diencephalon, Brainstem, and Ventricular System

The cerebral hemispheres of humans are so big that they cover over much of the rest of the CNS. The medial surface of a hemisected brain, however, reveals all the major divisions (Fig. 3-2), still arranged in the same sequence as in the embryonic neural tube: cerebral hemisphere-diencephalon-brainstem/cerebellum-spinal cord.

Two fiber bundles interconnect the cerebral hemispheres. The **corpus callosum** interconnects most cortical areas, extending from an enlarged **genu** in the

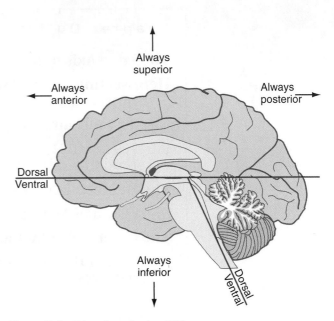

Figure 3-1   Directions in the CNS.

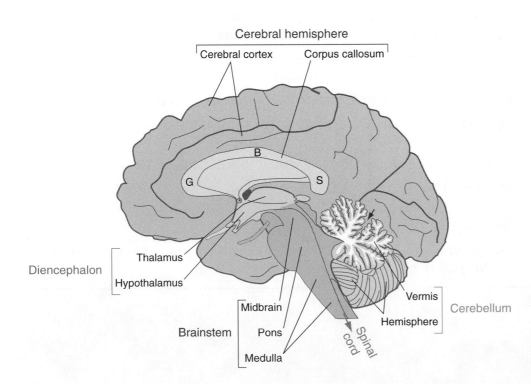

Figure 3-2   Major CNS subdivisions. *Arrow*, Primary fissure of the cerebellum; *, anterior commissure; *B, G, S,* body, genu, and splenium of the corpus callosum.

frontal lobe through a **body** to an enlarged **splenium** in the parietal lobe. The much smaller **anterior commissure** performs a similar function for parts of the temporal lobes. Beneath the corpus callosum in an accurately hemisected brain is a membrane called the **septum pellucidum**. This is a paired membrane (one per hemisphere) that separates those parts of the lateral ventricles adjacent to the midline (THB6 Figures 3-19 to 3-21, pp. 69 and 70). At the bottom of the septum pellucidum is the **fornix**, a long curved fiber bundle carrying the output of the **hippocampus** (see Fig. 3-6 later in this chapter) from the temporal lobe to structures like the hypothalamus at the base of the brain.

Hemisection passes through the middle of the third ventricle, exposing the thalamus and hypothalamus in its walls (Fig. 3-3). Each **interventricular foramen** connects the third ventricle to the lateral ventricle of that side. The **optic chiasm**, in which about half the fibers in each optic nerve cross the midline, is attached to the bottom of the hypothalamus. The **pineal gland** (part of the diencephalon) is attached to the roof of the third ventricle, near the diencephalon-brainstem junction.

The ventricular system continues through the midbrain as the cerebral aqueduct, then widens into the fourth ventricle of the pons and rostral medulla. The pons is characterized by a large basal portion (**basal pons**) that protrudes anteriorly.

The cerebellum is divided, in one gross anatomical sense, into a midline portion called the **vermis** (Latin for

"worm") and a much larger **hemisphere** on each side. In another gross anatomical sense, the deep **primary fissure** divides the bulk of the cerebellum into an **anterior lobe** and a substantially larger **posterior lobe**. Hence the anterior and posterior lobes have both vermal and hemispheral portions. Finally, there is a small **flocculonodular lobe**. The vermal part (the **nodulus**) can be seen in Fig. 3-3; the **flocculus** can be seen in THB6 Figures 3-16 and 3-17, pp. 65 and 66.

Named Sulci and Gyri Cover the Cerebral Surface

The surface of each cerebral hemisphere is wrinkled up into a series of **gyri** and **sulci**, constant from one brain to another in their general configuration but not in their details (THB6 Figure 3-6, p. 58). Four sulci are particularly important for defining the boundaries of cerebral lobes (Fig. 3-4)—the **lateral sulcus** (= **Sylvian fissure**) and **central sulcus** (of **Rolando**) on the lateral surface of the hemisphere, and the **parietooccipital** and **cingulate sulci** on the medial surface.

Each Cerebral Hemisphere Includes a Frontal, Parietal, Occipital, Temporal, and Limbic Lobe

Key Concepts

The frontal lobe contains motor areas.
The parietal lobe contains somatosensory areas.
The temporal lobe contains auditory areas.
The occipital lobe contains visual areas.
The limbic lobe is interconnected with other limbic structures buried in the temporal lobe.

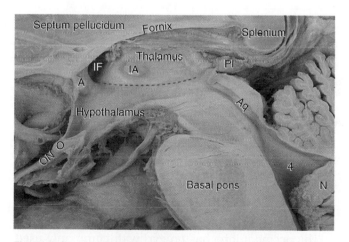

Figure 3-3 Parts of the diencephalon and nearby structures, seen in a hemisected brain. The *dashed line* indicates the shallow sulcus (hypothalamic sulcus) in the wall of the third ventricle that separates the thalamus and hypothalamus. *4,* Fourth ventricle; *A,* anterior commissure; *Aq,* cerebral aqueduct; *IA,* interthalamic adhesion (a gray matter connection between the two thalami, present in most but not all brains); *IF,* interventricular foramen; *N,* nodulus (part of the cerebellar vermis); *O,* optic chiasm; *ON,* optic nerve; *Pi,* pineal gland.

The **frontal lobe** is above the lateral sulcus and in front of the central sulcus. The **parietal lobe** is right behind the frontal lobe, extending back to the **occipital lobe** (which is defined by landmarks more easily visible on the medial surface of the hemisphere). The **temporal lobe** is below the lateral sulcus. All four of these lobes continue onto the medial surface of the hemisphere, extending as far as the **limbic lobe**. The limbic lobe is a ring of cortex that encircles the junction between the cerebral hemisphere and the diencephalon. In addition, the **insula**, not part of any of the preceding lobes, is buried in the lateral sulcus, covered over by parts of the frontal, parietal, and temporal lobes (see Fig. 2-6; and see THB6 Figure 3-8, p. 60).

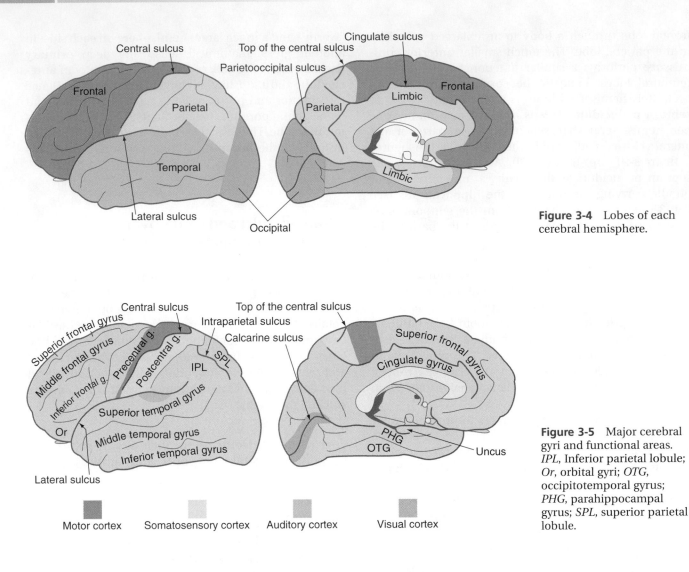

Figure 3-4 Lobes of each cerebral hemisphere.

Figure 3-5 Major cerebral gyri and functional areas. *IPL*, Inferior parietal lobule; *Or*, orbital gyri; *OTG*, occipitotemporal gyrus; *PHG*, parahippocampal gyrus; *SPL*, superior parietal lobule.

The lateral surface of the frontal lobe is made up of the **precentral gyrus** and the **superior**, **middle**, and **inferior frontal gyri** (Fig. 3-5). The precentral gyrus is located immediately in front of the central sulcus and most of it is **primary motor cortex** (i.e., much of the corticospinal tract originates here). The other three are broad, parallel gyri that extend anteriorly from the precentral gyrus. The precentral and superior frontal gyri extend over onto the medial surface of the frontal lobe, where they end at the cingulate sulcus. The inferior (or **orbital**) surface of the frontal lobe is made up of a series of unnamed orbital gyri together with **gyrus rectus**, which is located adjacent to the midline.

The major named gyrus of the parietal lobe is the **postcentral gyrus**. The postcentral gyrus corresponds to **primary somatosensory cortex** (i.e., ascending somatosensory pathways terminate most heavily here) and, like the precentral gyrus, extends over onto the medial surface of the parietal lobe. The rest of the lateral surface is occupied by the **superior** and **inferior**

parietal lobules, separated by the deep **intraparietal sulcus**.

The temporal lobe is covered by four long, parallel gyri. The **superior**, **middle**, and **inferior temporal gyri** are exposed on the lateral surface. The inferior temporal gyrus extends around onto the inferior surface and is followed by the **occipitotemporal gyrus**. Most **primary auditory cortex** is located in transverse temporal gyri in the wall of the lateral sulcus; it extends laterally to occupy a small portion of the superior temporal gyrus.

The occipital lobe has no gyri with commonly used names. However, its medial surface is bisected by the **calcarine sulcus**. **Primary visual cortex** occupies the walls of this sulcus and extends out onto the medial surface.

The major components of the limbic lobe are the **cingulate** and **parahippocampal gyri**. The cingulate gyrus curves around adjacent to the corpus callosum, interposed between it and the frontal and parietal lobes. Near the splenium of the corpus callosum the cingulate gyrus is continuous with the parahippocampal gyrus, which proceeds parallel to the occipitotemporal gyrus. At its anterior end the parahippocampal gyrus folds back on itself to form a bump called the **uncus**. The parahippocampal gyrus received its name because it is continuous with a cortical region called the **hippocampus**, which is rolled into the interior of the hemisphere and visible only in sections (see Fig. 3-6).

The Diencephalon Includes the Thalamus and Hypothalamus

Key Concepts

The thalamus conveys information to the cerebral cortex.
The hypothalamus controls the autonomic nervous system.

Each region of the diencephalon contains the term "thalamus" in its name. The **epithalamus** includes the pineal gland and a few other small structures. The **subthalamus**, completely surrounded by other parts of the CNS, includes an important component of the basal ganglia (see Chapter 19). The thalamus and hypothalamus form the walls of the third ventricle. Most pathways headed for the cerebral cortex involve a synapse in the thalamus (see Chapter 16), which controls access to the cortex. The hypothalamus (see Chapter 23) controls the autonomic nervous system and gets involved in various aspects of drive-related behaviors.

Most Cranial Nerves Are Attached to the Brainstem

The brainstem has three longitudinal subdivisions: the midbrain (continuous with the diencephalon), pons, and medulla (continuous with the spinal cord).

Most of the brainstem's general functions you could probably guess. **Cranial nerves III–XII** attach here (THB6 Figure 3-17, p. 66), and the brainstem is concerned with processing their incoming information (and sending it on to the thalamus), with **cranial nerve reflexes** (e.g., you blink when something touches your cornea), and with getting motor commands out through cranial nerves. A second general kind of function has to do with the fact that the brainstem is interposed between the cerebrum and the spinal cord. That means that a spinothalamic tract or a corticospinal tract would need to traverse the brainstem. These are usually

referred to as the **long tract functions** of the brainstem. Finally, and one which you wouldn't necessarily have guessed, the brainstem has some more global functions of its own. For example, it's got some built-in circuitry (the **Ascending Reticular Activating System**) that regulates our state of consciousness and is central to the sleep-wake cycle.

The Cerebellum Includes a Vermis and Two Hemispheres

There are several different ways to divide up the cerebellum (see Chapter 20), but subdividing it into longitudinal strips (i.e., perpendicular to the mostly transverse sulci and fissures) corresponds best to the way the cerebellum is wired up functionally. On a gross level, the whole cerebellum can be divided into a longitudinal midline strip called the vermis (mostly concerned with coordinating trunk movements), flanked on each side by a cerebellar hemisphere (mostly concerned with coordinating limb movements).

Sections of the Cerebrum Reveal the Basal Ganglia and Limbic Structures

Key Concepts

Many parts of each cerebral hemisphere are arranged in a C shape.
The caudate nucleus, putamen, and globus pallidus are major components of the basal ganglia.
The amygdala and hippocampus are major limbic structures.

A number of forebrain structures are completely enveloped by the cerebral hemispheres and cannot be seen without sectioning the brain (Fig. 3-6). Coronal sections reveal the general arrangement of these structures; horizontal sections help to reveal their extent.

Two major components of the basal ganglia, the **putamen** and the **globus pallidus** (referred to together as the **lenticular nucleus**), lie beneath the insula. Another major forebrain component of the basal ganglia, the **caudate** ("having a tail") **nucleus**, follows the wall of the lateral ventricle. Like the lateral ventricle, the caudate nucleus is C-shaped. It extends from an enlarged **head** in the frontal lobe, through a **body** in the frontal and parietal lobes, to a thin **tail** in the temporal lobe.

A thick bundle of fibers called the **internal capsule** runs between the lenticular nucleus and the thalamus; it continues anteriorly between the lenticular nucleus

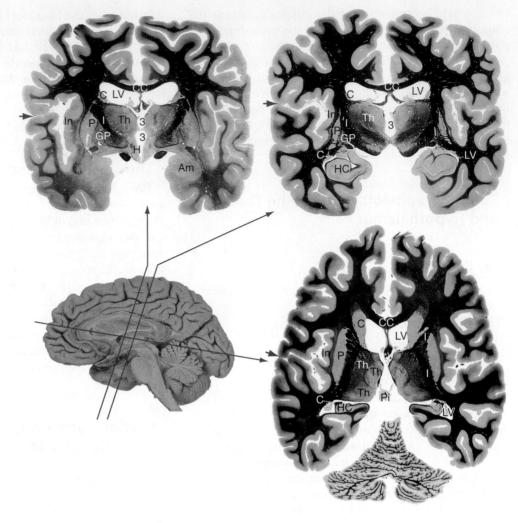

Figure 3-6 Major structures inside the cerebrum. *Red arrows* indicate the lateral sulcus, leading to the insula (In). *, Fornix; *3*, third ventricle; *Am*, amygdala; *C*, caudate nucleus; *CC*, corpus callosum; *GP*, globus pallidus; *H*, hypothalamus; *HC*, hippocampus; *I*, internal capsule; *LV*, lateral ventricle; *P*, putamen; *Pi*, pineal gland: *Th*, thalamus.

and the head of the caudate nucleus. The internal capsule is the principal route through which fibers travel between the cerebral cortex and subcortical sites. For example, the corticospinal tract travels through the internal capsule, as do somatosensory fibers from the thalamus to the cortex.

Underlying the uncus in the more anterior of the two coronal sections in Figure 3-6 is a large nucleus called the **amygdala**, an important component of the limbic system. Just posterior to it, in the other coronal section, is the most anterior part of the **hippocampus**, a cortical structure that has been folded into the temporal lobe. The hippocampus is another major component of the limbic system.

Parts of the Nervous System Are Interconnected in Systematic Ways

Neural pathways can look pretty complicated, but there are in fact some wiring principles that often apply. Each

of them has exceptions, but collectively they can make the connection patterns easier to understand.

Axons of Primary Afferents and Lower Motor Neurons Convey Information to and from the CNS

> **Key Concepts**
>
> Axons of primary afferents enter the CNS without crossing the midline.
> Axons of lower motor neurons leave the CNS without crossing the midline.

The CNS communicates with the rest of the body primarily through sensory neurons and motor neurons. **Primary afferent neurons** convey information into the CNS; some have specialized receptive endings outside the CNS and others have peripheral endings that receive connections from separate **receptor cells**. Primary afferents typically have their cell bodies in ganglia adjacent to the CNS, and central processes that synapse in the CNS. (A CNS neuron on which a primary afferent synapses is called a **second order neuron**, which in turn synapses on a **third order neuron**, etc.) With few exceptions, the receptive endings, cell body, and central terminals of primary afferents are all on the same side (Fig. 3-7). Motor neurons that innervate skeletal muscle (also called **lower motor neurons**) have their cell bodies within the CNS but, like primary afferents, they are almost always connected to **ipsilateral** structures.

Somatosensory Inputs Participate in Reflexes, Pathways to the Cerebellum, and Pathways to the Cerebral Cortex

Most kinds of sensory information divide into three streams after entering the CNS (Fig. 3-8), each stream usually being actually a series of parallel creeks. The first stream feeds into local reflex pathways, the second is directed to the cerebral cortex, and the third to the cerebellum. The information that reaches the cerebral cortex is used in our conscious awareness of the world, as well as in figuring out appropriate behavioral responses to what's going on out there. The information that reaches the cerebellum, in contrast, is used in motor control; someone with cerebellar dysfunction moves abnormally but has normal awareness of the abnormal movements.

We have only one set of primary afferents, and each of them has numerous branches in the CNS that collectively lead to all of these streams. So each fiber coming from a muscle stretch receptor, for example, has branches that feed into reflex arcs, others that feed into pathways to the cerebral cortex, and still others that feed into pathways to the cerebellum.

Somatosensory Pathways to the Cerebral Cortex Cross the Midline and Pass through the Thalamus

Somatosensory pathways to the cerebral cortex contain at least three neurons (some contain more): a primary afferent, a second order neuron that projects to the thalamus, and a third order neuron that projects from the thalamus to the cortex. In the case of somatic sensation, one side of the body is represented in the cerebral cortex of the opposite side. Because neither primary afferents nor thalamocortical neurons have axons that cross the midline, it follows that second order neurons are the ones with crossing axons. One key to understanding

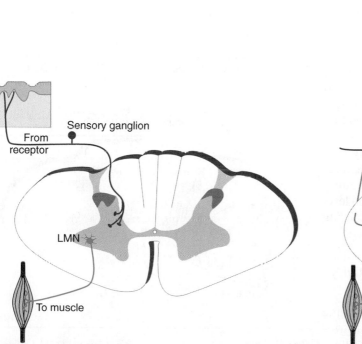

Figure 3-7   Primary afferents and lower motor neurons (*LMN*).

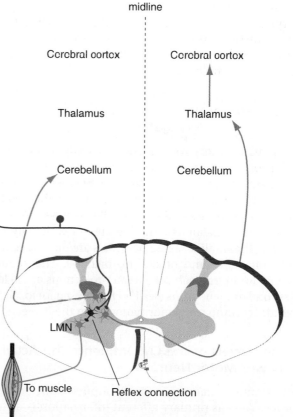

Figure 3-8   Distribution of somatosensory information. *LMN*, Lower motor neuron.

the organization of sensory pathways is knowing the location of the second order neurons (THB6 Figure 3-29, p. 76).

Somatosensory Cortex Contains a Distorted Map of the Body

A recurring theme in the CNS is systematic mapping—in the cortex and even in cross sections of pathways, adjacent areas or adjacent fibers represent neighboring parts of the body, or contiguous places in the visual field, or successive sound frequencies. The maps are usually distorted, emphasizing areas where we have high acuity or fine control. For example, one reason we can use our fingertips for high-acuity tasks like reading Braille is that fingertips contain lots of receptive endings. So there are lots of fibers representing the fingers in somatosensory pathways, as well as a large area in somatosensory cortex where the fingers are represented (THB6 Figure 3-30, p. 76).

Each Side of the Cerebellum Receives Information about the Ipsilateral Side of the Body

Pathways from the periphery to the cerebellum are simpler, because the thalamus is not involved. At their simplest, they contain only a primary afferent and a second order neuron that projects to the cerebellum. Curiously, one side of the cerebellum is related to the same side of the body. Part of the basis for this situation is that sensory pathways to the cerebellum typically do not cross the midline.

Other Sensory Systems Are Similar to the Somatosensory System

The somatosensory system is representative in most ways of sensory systems in general. Other systems feed into reflex arcs, reach the cerebellum, have distorted maps, and take at least three neurons to reach the cerebral cortex. (The only exception is the olfactory system, which bypasses the thalamus). The big area of variability is in crossing the midline; some pathways are uncrossed (e.g., taste, olfaction) and others are bilateral. The auditory system, for example, has bilateral projections at the level of second order neurons (see Fig. 14-5), used for localizing sounds by comparing information from the two ears.

Higher Levels of the CNS Influence the Activity of Lower Motor Neurons

Lower motor neurons receive inputs from multiple sources (just as primary afferent information is distributed to multiple places). There are more details in Chapters 10 and 18-20, but basically, the sources are **upper motor neurons** in the cerebral cortex and brainstem, together with local reflex connections. The cerebellum and basal ganglia also affect lower motor neurons, but not directly.

Corticospinal Axons Cross the Midline

Signals for the initiation of voluntary movements issue from the cerebral cortex. The thalamus is not a relay in pathways *leaving* the cerebral cortex, and there is a large **corticospinal tract** that projects directly from cortex to spinal cord (and an analogous **corticobulbar tract** that projects to cranial nerve motor nuclei). Most corticospinal fibers, consistent with the pattern in the somatosensory system, cross the midline (Fig. 3-9).

Just as some sensory systems project bilaterally to the thalamus and cortex, some motor neurons receive bilateral innervation from the cerebral cortex. This is particularly true of motor neurons for muscles near the midline that normally work together, such as the muscles of the larynx and pharynx. Motor neurons to limb muscles, on the other hand, receive an almost entirely crossed corticospinal innervation.

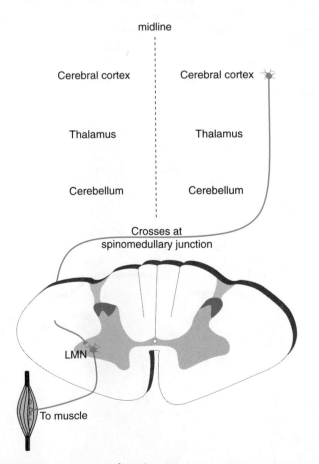

Figure 3-9 Crossing of corticospinal axons. *LMN*, Lower motor neuron.

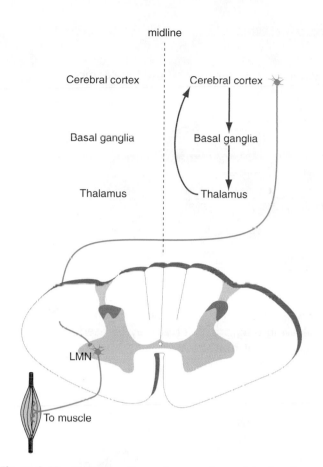

Figure 3-10 General pattern of connections of the basal ganglia. *LMN*, Lower motor neuron.

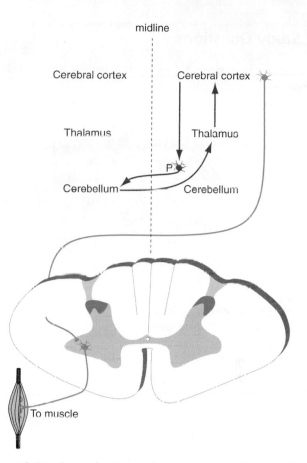

Figure 3-11 General pattern of connections of the cerebellum with the cerebrum. *LMN*, Lower motor neuron; *P*, neuron in the basal pons.

The Basal Ganglia and Cerebellum Indirectly Affect Contralateral and Ipsilateral Motor Neurons, Respectively

The basal ganglia and the cerebellum are also involved in control of movement. However, both work not by influencing motor neurons directly, but mostly by affecting the output of motor areas of the cortex. Connections between the basal ganglia and the cerebral cortex for the most part do not cross the midline (Fig. 3-10), so one-sided damage to the basal ganglia causes **contralateral** deficits. In contrast, connections between the cerebrum and the cerebellum are crossed (Fig. 3-11), consistent with the observation that one-sided cerebellar damage causes ipsilateral deficits. Because the cerebellum and basal ganglia affect motor but not sensory areas of the cortex, damage to the cerebellum or basal ganglia does not cause changes in basic sensation.

Study Questions

Answer questions 1-5 using the letters on the following diagram. A letter may be used once, more than once, or not at all.

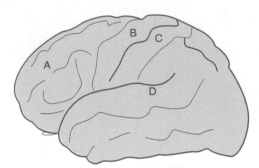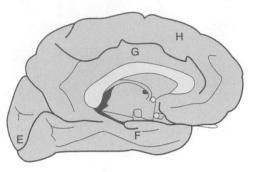

1. Somatosensory cortex
2. Superior frontal gyrus
3. Part of the parietal lobe
4. Visual cortex
5. Parahippocampal gyrus

Answer questions 6-10 using the letters on the following diagram. A letter may be used once, more than once, or not at all.

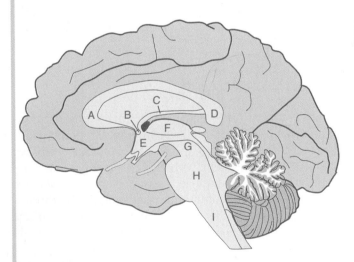

Answer questions 11-15 using the letters on the following diagram. A letter may be used once, more than once, or not at all.

6. Pons
7. Splenium of the corpus callosum
8. Output from the hippocampus
9. Major relay in pathways to the cerebral cortex
10. Control center for the autonomic nervous system

11. Insula
12. Lenticular nucleus
13. Thalamus
14. Part of the basal ganglia
15. Hippocampus

Study Questions—cont'd

16. The primary afferent neurons for touch in the big toe have their cell bodies in
    a. ipsilateral spinal gray matter.
    b. contralateral spinal gray matter.
    c. ipsilateral ganglia adjacent to the spinal cord.
    d. contralateral ganglia adjacent to the spinal cord.

17. The facial nerve controls the muscles used to wrinkle the forehead, as well as those used for smiling. Damage to motor cortex on one side commonly causes weakness of contralateral smiling muscles but does not cause pronounced weakness of forehead muscles on either side. The most likely explanation of this observation is that
    a. each facial motor nucleus has motor neurons for the forehead muscles of both sides, but the smiling muscles of only one side.
    b. the cerebral cortex of each side sends mostly crossed projections to some facial motor neurons, and bilateral projections to other facial motor neurons.

18. Damage to a sensory area of the left cerebral cortex causes deficits on the right because
    a. primary afferents cross the midline on their way to second-order cells.
    b. second-order cells have axons that cross the midline on the way to the thalamus.
    c. thalamic neurons project to the contralateral cerebral cortex.
    d. any of the above could be responsible, depending on the sensory system involved.

19. Damage to the right side of the cerebellum causes
    a. incoordination of the right arm due to inability to perceive its position.
    b. incoordination of the left arm due to inability to perceive its position.
    c. difficulty controlling the left arm, with full awareness of its abnormal movement.
    d. difficulty controlling the right arm, with full awareness of its abnormal movement.

20. Damage to the right basal ganglia causes a left-sided movement disorder because
    a. fibers from the basal ganglia descend to the spinal cord, crossing along the way.
    b. fibers from the basal ganglia project to the contralateral thalamus, which in turn projects to the spinal cord.
    c. fibers from the basal ganglia project to the ipsilateral thalamus, which in turn sends crossed fibers to the spinal cord.
    d. the basal ganglia project to the thalamus, which in turn projects to motor cortex; these connections are all uncrossed, but motor cortex sends crossed fibers to the spinal cord.

Meningeal Coverings of the Brain and Spinal Cord

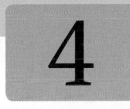

Chapter Outline

The meninges form a major part of the mechanical suspension system of the CNS, necessary to keep it from self-destructing as we move through the world. In addition, one layer of the meninges participates in the system of barriers that effectively isolates the extracellular spaces in the nervous system from the extracellular spaces in the rest of the body.

mater (or **pia**) are much thinner collagenous membranes. The arachnoid is attached to the inside of the dura and the pia is attached to the outer surface of the CNS. Hence the only space normally present between or around the cranial meninges is **subarachnoid space** (not counting the **venous sinuses** found within the dura). The arrangement of spinal meninges is slightly different, as described later in this chapter.

There Are Three Meningeal Layers: The Dura Mater, Arachnoid, and Pia Mater

The **dura mater**, or **dura**, is a thick connective tissue membrane that also serves as the periosteum of the inside of the skull (Fig. 4-1). The **arachnoid** and the **pia**

The Dura Mater Provides Mechanical Strength

The thickness and abundant collagen of the dura make it the mechanical link that connects the skull to the deli-

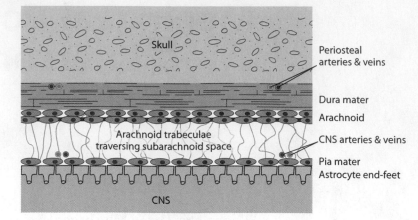

Figure 4-1 Overview of the meninges. The dark bars interconnecting the innermost arachnoid cells indicate the bands of tight junctions that form the arachnoid barrier.

cate strands of arachnoid (**arachnoid trabeculae**) that suspend the CNS in its bath of cerebrospinal fluid (CSF). This combination of partial flotation of the CNS in subarachnoid CSF, together with mechanical suspension by the skull-dura-arachnoid-arachnoid trabeculae-pia-CNS connections (see Fig. 4-3), stabilizes the fragile CNS during routine head movements.

Dural Septa Partially Separate Different Intracranial Compartments

The skull-dura-CNS suspension just described would not prevent different brain parts (e.g., the two cerebral hemispheres, or the cerebellum and the occipital lobes) from slapping against each other during head movements. This is addressed by sheetlike extensions of the dura that form **dural reflections** or **dural septa**, carrying the suspension system inward. The two most prominent of these are the **falx cerebri**, separating the two cerebral hemispheres, and the **tentorium cerebelli**, separating the cerebellum and brainstem (below it) from the forebrain (above it). These can't be complete separations because the two cerebral hemispheres are interconnected beneath the falx by the corpus callosum, and the brainstem continues upward through the **tentorial notch** into the diencephalon. The free edges of these dural reflections are sites at which expanding masses can cause **herniation** of part of the brain from one compartment into another (THB6 Figure 4-19, p. 96).

The Dura Mater Contains Venous Sinuses That Drain the Brain

Along attached edges of dural reflections (and along some free edges) there is an endothelium-lined venous channel within the dura, called a **dural venous sinus**. Prominent sinuses are the **superior sagittal sinus** (along the attachment of the falx cerebri to the skull), left and right **transverse sinuses** (along the attachment of the tentorium cerebelli to the skull), and the **straight sinus** (along the attachment of the falx and tentorium to each other). All four meet at the back of the head in the **confluence of the sinuses** (also called the **torcular**, or torcular Herophili, Greek for "the winepress of Herophilus"). Venous drainage from the brain eventually reaches these sinuses (THB6 Figure 6-31, p.144).

The Dura Mater Has Its Own Blood Supply

In addition to the venous sinuses that drain the brain, the dura contains a mostly separate set of arteries and veins that help with its periosteal role for the skull (see Fig. 4-1). **Meningeal arteries** can be important clinically because tearing one can cause bleeding between the skull and dura (epidural bleeding, described later).

The Dura Mater Is Pain Sensitive

The dura and some subarachnoid blood vessels are the only pain-sensitive intracranial structures. So inflammation (e.g., meningitis) or traction (e.g., by an expanding mass) causes headache. The brain itself has no pain-sensitive endings.

The Dura Mater Has an Arachnoid Lining

The arachnoid is attached to the skull by virtue of its attachment to the dura. The pia is attached to the CNS. Hence, the arachnoid trabeculae that interconnect the pia and arachnoid form a relatively weak mechanical suspension system for the CNS. The CNS is completely immersed in the CSF that fills subarachnoid space. The partial flotation effect of this CSF reduces the effective weight of the CNS to the point that the meningeal suspension system can support the brain and spinal cord (see Fig. 4-3).

The Arachnoid Bridges over CNS Surface Irregularities, Forming Cisterns

Subarachnoid space is filled with CSF, contains the arteries and veins that supply and drain the CNS, and is traversed by arachnoid trabeculae. Large pockets of subarachnoid space, corresponding to major irregularities in the surface of the CNS, are called **subarachnoid cisterns** (THB6 Figure 4-10, p. 00). Prominent intracranial cisterns include **cisterna magna** (between the medulla and the inferior surface of the cerebellum) and the **superior cistern** (above the midbrain).

CSF Enters the Venous Circulation through Arachnoid Villi

Arachnoid outpouchings poke through holes in the walls of venous sinuses as **arachnoid villi** (Fig. 4-2). Here only an arachnoid layer and an endothelial layer separate CSF and venous blood, the arachnoid barrier (see next section) is missing, and CSF can move directly from subarachnoid space into venous blood. Arachnoid villi act like mechanical flap valves, so when CSF pressure is higher than venous pressure (the usual situation), CSF moves into the venous system. If the reverse situation occurs, the villi snap shut and venous blood doesn't enter subarachnoid space.

The Arachnoid Has a Barrier Function

The arachnoid includes a layer of cells that are connected to each other by bands of tight junctions, represented by dark bars in Figs. 4-1 and 4-2. This forms a barrier to the diffusion of extracellular substances from the dura into CSF, or in the reverse direction. The **arachnoid barrier** is part of a system, summarized in Chapter 6, that effectively separates the extracellular fluids of the nervous system from those of the rest of the body.

Pia Mater Covers the Surface of the CNS

The thin pia mater is attached on one side to arachnoid trabeculae and on the other to the astrocyte end-feet that carpet the surface of the CNS. This completes the mechanical suspension system.

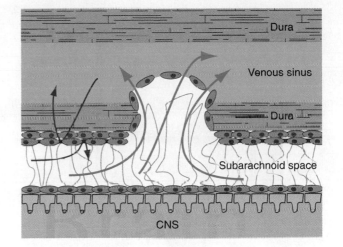

Figure 4-2 Arachnoid barrier and villus. CSF can pour through functional holes in each arachnoid villus to reach venous blood, but solutes are unable to cross the arachnoid at other sites.

The Vertebral Canal Contains Spinal Epidural Space

Spinal meninges are similar in principle to cranial meninges: thick dura lined by arachnoid, subarachnoid space filled with CSF, and suspensory interconnections between arachnoid and pia (Fig. 4-3). However, at the level of the foramen magnum the periosteal component of the cranial dura continues around onto the outer surface of the skull. The result is a real **spinal epidural space** between the spinal dura and the vertebral periosteum (as opposed to the *potential* cranial epidural space, which when present is located between the periosteum and the skull).

Arachnoid trabeculae are thickened around the spinal cord to form **denticulate ligaments**. The spinal cord is shorter than the vertebral canal (see Chapter 10), so there's a large subarachnoid cistern, the **lumbar cistern**, extending from vertebral levels L1/L2 to S2.

Bleeding Can Open Up Potential Meningeal Spaces

Key Concepts

Tearing of meningeal arteries can cause an epidural hematoma.
Tearing of veins where they enter venous sinuses can cause a subdural hematoma.

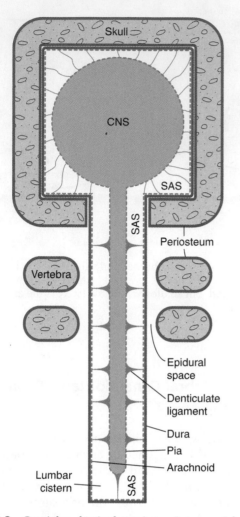

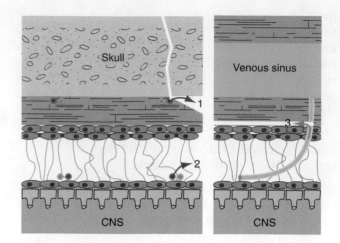

Figure 4-4 Bleeding into real and potential meningeal spaces. Tearing a meningeal artery, typically as the result of a skull fracture, causes epidural bleeding (*1*). Rupture of a cerebral artery, as in a burst aneurysm, causes subarachnoid bleeding (*2*). Tearing a cerebral vein as it penetrates the arachnoid (*3*) on its way into a venous sinus causes subdural bleeding (that actually separates the innermost layers of the dura).

Figure 4-3 Cranial and spinal meninges. Intracranial dura is, in effect, double-layered; the periosteal layer continues onto the outside of the skull, leaving a single-layered spinal dural sheath separated from vertebral periosteum by a real epidural space. SAS, subarachnoid space.

Spaces are not normally present between the dura and either the skull or the arachnoid, but these **potential epidural** and **subdural* spaces** can be opened up in certain pathological conditions (Fig. 4-4; see THB6 Figure 4-14, p. 92). Most often this is caused by tearing of a meningeal artery (leading to epidural bleeding) or of a cerebral vein as it enters a dural venous sinus (leading to subdural bleeding). Rupture of ordinary cerebral arteries and veins causes subarachnoid bleeding

because these vessels reside in subarachnoid space. Each has a characteristic appearance in clinical images: Epidural hematomas are usually localized and lens-shaped (THB6 Figure 4-15, p. 93), subdural hematomas are usually larger and crescent-shaped (THB6 Figure 4-18, p. 95), and subarachnoid bleeding fills sulci and cisterns (THB6 Figure 6-25, p. 141).

Parts of the CNS Can Herniate from One Intracranial Compartment into Another

Because the dural septa are tough and taut, and brain is soft and squishy, expanding masses (e.g., hematomas, tumors) can cause parts of the brain to herniate from one side of a dural septum to another (THB6 Figure 4-19, p. 96). The most common such herniations are for one cingulate gyrus to herniate under the falx, or (more ominously) for the uncus of one temporal lobe to herniate through the tentorial notch and compress the midbrain. Similarly, an expanding mass in the posterior fossa can cause low-hanging parts of the cerebellum (the **cerebellar tonsils**; see Fig. 20-1) to herniate through the foramen magnum and compress the medulla.

---

*Although conventionally referred to as subdural space, the splitting actually occurs in the innermost part of the dura.

Study Questions

1. A 39-year-old handball player collided with a wall while running full speed and hit the left side of his head. He became progressively more disoriented and lethargic over the next 2 hours and was taken to the emergency department. Imaging studies revealed a skull fracture, a torn middle meningeal artery, and an expanding hematoma compressing the left side of his brain. This bleeding was most likely to have occurred in the
    a. epidural space.
    b. intradural space.
    c. subdural space.
    d. subarachnoid space.
    e. subpial space.

2. Real spaces within the cranium include
    a. subdural space.
    b. subarachnoid space.
    c. epidural space.
    d. a and b.
    e. none of the above.

3. The thickest, mechanically strongest part of the meninges is the
    a. dura mater.
    b. arachnoid.
    c. pia mater.

4. A mass in one parietal lobe might cause the ipsilateral cingulate gyrus to herniate
    a. under the falx cerebri.
    b. through the tentorial notch.
    c. past the tentorium cerebelli.
    d. through the foramen magnum.

5. A small protein molecule located in the periosteum of the skull and diffusing toward the brain would meet a diffusion barrier
    a. in the dura mater.
    b. in a layer of arachnoid cells
    c. in the pia mater.
    d. nowhere.

6. Cerebrospinal fluid moves into venous blood by
    a. diffusing through the dural walls of venous sinuses.
    b. being actively transported across the arachnoid
    c. passing through functional holes in the arachnoid villi.
    d. passing directly across the walls of veins in subarachnoid space.

7. Which of the following is least important in the maintenance of the shape and position of the CNS?
    a. arachnoid trabeculae.
    b. denticulate ligaments.
    c. mechanical rigidity of the CNS.
    d. partial flotation effect of the cerebrospinal fluid in subarachnoid space.
    e. physical attachment of the arachnoid to the dura.

8. One characteristic of the meninges of the spinal cord is
    a. real epidural space, between the dura and the vertebral periosteum.
    b. potential epidural space, between dura and vertebral periosteum.
    c. no subarachnoid space.
    d. real subdural space.

Ventricles and Cerebrospinal Fluid

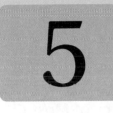

The **ventricular system**, the remnant of the space in the middle of the embryonic neural tube (see Fig. 2-5), is an interconnected series of cavities that extends through most of the CNS.

The Brain Contains Four Ventricles

There's a pair of **lateral ventricles** in the telencephalon (one for each cerebral hemisphere), a midline **third ventricle** in the diencephalon, and a **fourth ventricle** that straddles the midline in the pons and medulla. **Cerebrospinal fluid** (CSF) is secreted within the ventricles, fills them, and flows out of the fourth ventricle through three apertures to fill subarachnoid space.

A Lateral Ventricle Curves through Each Cerebral Hemisphere

Each lateral ventricle is basically a C-shaped structure. This C shape curves from an **inferior horn** in the temporal lobe through a **body** in the parietal lobe and a bit of the frontal lobe, ending at the **interventricular foramen** where each lateral ventricle joins the third ventricle. Along this C-shaped course two extensions emerge—a **posterior horn** that extends backward into the occipital lobe and an **anterior horn** that extends farther into the frontal lobe (Fig. 5-1; see THB6 Figure 5-2, p. 101). The expanded area where the body and the inferior and posterior horns meet is called the **atrium**. Each lateral ventricle represents the cavity of an embryonic telencephalic vesicle, so telencephalic structures

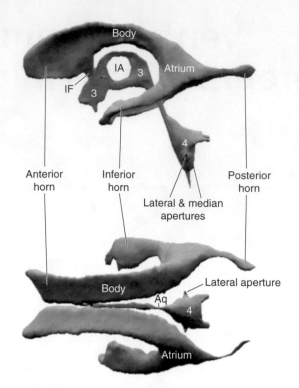

Figure 5-1   The ventricles. *3*, Third ventricle; *4*, fourth ventricle; *Aq*, aqueduct; *IA*, interthalamic adhesion; *IF*, interventricular foramen. *(Thanks to Dr. John Sundsten.)*

like the caudate nucleus and the hippocampus border much of it; the thalamus, a diencephalic derivative, also forms part of its floor (THB6 Figures 3-19 to 3-24, pp. 69-71).

The Third Ventricle Is a Midline Cavity in the Diencephalon

The third ventricle is a midline slit in the diencephalon, with walls formed by the hypothalamus and much of the thalamus. The thalamus grows right across the third ventricle in most human brains, forming an **interthalamic adhesion**, so that the ventricle winds up looking like a misshapen doughnut.

The Fourth Ventricle Communicates with Subarachnoid Cisterns

The fourth ventricle extends from the **cerebral aqueduct** of the midbrain, through which it communicates with the third ventricle, to a mid-medullary level, where it narrows down into the vestigial **central canal** of the caudal medulla and the spinal cord. It reaches its widest extent at the pontomedullary junction, where it extends into a **lateral recess** on each side. The tent-like roof of the fourth ventricle pokes up into the cerebellum.

The ventricular system communicates with subarachnoid space through three apertures of the fourth ventricle, a **lateral aperture** at the end of each lateral recess and a **median aperture** above the point where the fourth ventricle narrows down into the central canal.

The Ventricles Contain Only a Fraction of the CSF

Although CSF is made in the ventricles, most of it is physically located in subarachnoid space (about 25 mL in the ventricles vs. 150 mL or so in subarachnoid space).

Choroid Plexus Is the Source of Most CSF

> **Key Concept**
>
> The ependymal lining of choroid plexus is specialized as a secretory epithelium.

Choroid plexus is formed at certain areas where the inner lining (i.e., ependyma) and the outer covering (i.e., pia) of the CNS are directly applied to each other, with no intervening neural tissue. At these sites, the ependymal cells are specialized as a secretory epithelium called **choroid epithelium**; adjacent cells are joined by tight junctions, forming a diffusion barrier. Vascular connective tissue invaginates this pia/ependyma membrane, forming multiply folded choroid plexus (Fig. 5-2). This means that wherever you see choroid plexus, one side faces a ventricle and the other side faces subarachnoid space (THB6 Figure 5-8, p. 106).

A long strand of choroid plexus follows the C shape of each lateral ventricle, grows through the interventricular foramen, and joins the roof of the third ventricle (THB6 Figure 5-7, p. 105). Separate strands of choroid plexus grow in the roof of the fourth ventricle, extending laterally through the lateral apertures and caudally to the median aperture.

CSF Is a Secretion of the Choroid Plexus

Capillaries in choroid plexus, unlike most other capillaries inside the arachnoid barrier, are permeable to plasma solutes. Plasma solutes therefore leak out, cross the pial layer, get stopped by the choroid epithelial diffusion barrier, and form the substrate for active secretion of CSF into the ventricles by the choroid epithelium. The

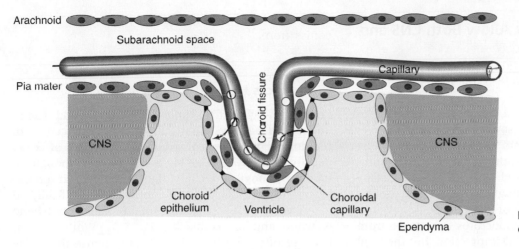

Figure 5-2 Composition of choroid plexus.

resulting CSF is clear and colorless, low in protein, and similar (but not identical) to serum in its ionic composition.

CSF Circulates through and around the CNS, Eventually Reaching the Venous System

The cerebrospinal fluid secreted by the choroid plexuses moves through the ventricular system (Fig. 5-3), pushed along by newly formed CSF. It leaves the fourth ventricle through the lateral and median apertures, moves through subarachnoid space until it reaches the arachnoid villi (most of which protrude into the superior sagittal sinus), and finally joins the venous circulation (Fig. 5-4).

Movement across the arachnoid villi is passive, driven by the difference in hydrostatic pressure between the CSF in subarachnoid space and the venous blood in the superior sagittal sinus. The villi act like tiny flap valves so that reverse flow is prevented if venous pressure exceeds CSF pressure.

CSF Has Multiple Functions

CSF has two general kinds of functions—some physical and some chemical. The major physical functions are that (1) the CNS nearly floats in subarachnoid CSF, making it easier for the meninges to stabilize the CNS inside the head and spine, and (2) CSF is a spatial buffer and some can be squeezed out of the head to make way for things like arterial pulses (THB6 Figure 5-11, p. 109). The chemical functions are based on the free diffusion between CSF and the extracellular fluids around neurons; this means that CSF changes (e.g., changes in ionic concentrations or hormone levels) will reach neurons.

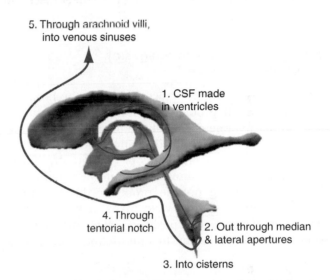

Figure 5-3 Circulation of CSF. CSF emerges from the fourth ventricle into the posterior fossa, so most of it has to flow through the tentorial notch, alongside the brainstem, to reach arachnoid villi in the superior sagittal and other sinuses. *(Thanks to Dr. John Sundsten.)*

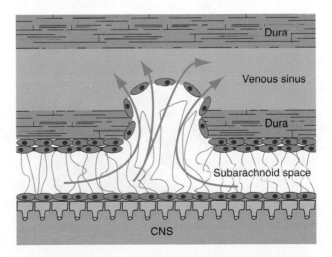

Figure 5-4 Movement of CSF through an arachnoid villus.

Imaging Techniques Allow Both CNS and CSF To Be Visualized

There are two big problems in trying to make pictures of the brains of live, unopened people. One is generating contrast (i.e., getting skull, blood, CSF, and brain to yield different amounts of some signal). The other is getting a 3D impression from a 2D picture. For a long time both problems were approached somewhat indirectly. Contrast was produced where it doesn't usually exist, for example by getting air into the ventricles (**pneumoencephalography**) or x-ray dense liquids into blood vessels (**angiography**). Pictures were taken from multiple angles to create a 3D impression, but they still involved flattening all the contrast in a solid object into a 2D picture.

Tomography Produces Images of 2-Dimensional "Slices"

Constructing pictures of "slices" through the head can get around both problems: plotting x-ray density or some other parameter in a single plane prevents some areas from swamping out, or being superimposed on, others. There are several kinds of tomography, but all depend on basically similar computer-assisted calculations. Depending on the probe or the measuring device, the process may yield maps of x-ray density, water concentration, positron concentration, or something else. The key to interpreting tomographic images lies in understanding where the contrast comes from.

CT Produces Maps of X-Ray Density

Rotating x-ray sources and detectors around someone's head and systematically varying the center of rotation allows the construction of maps of x-ray density (THB6 Figure 5-14, p. 112). (Even though all modern **tomography** is a variant of computed tomography, folks usually use the term CT specifically to mean **x-ray CT**.) Just as with plain skull x-rays, bone is white and air is black (Fig. 5-5). White matter, because of all the lipid, is less x-ray dense than gray matter and so is darker; CSF, which is mostly water, is darker still.

MRI Produces Maps of Water Concentration

Magnetic resonance imaging (**MRI**) is based on similar calculations but a fundamentally different signal—the re-emission of radio waves absorbed by atoms in a strong magnetic field. The most abundant source of such signals in the CNS is protons, mostly in water but also in other molecules. Because the free water concentration and the concentrations of other molecules varies in different parts of the CNS and adjoining areas, white matter, gray matter, and CSF all look different. Different time constants can be used to produce images

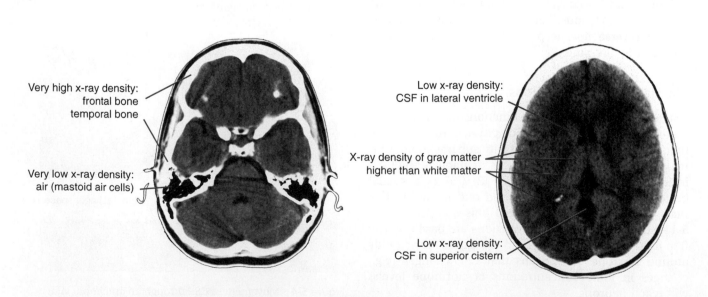

Very high x-ray density:
frontal bone
temporal bone

Very low x-ray density:
air (mastoid air cells)

Low x-ray density:
CSF in lateral ventricle

X-ray density of gray matter
higher than white matter

Low x-ray density:
CSF in superior cistern

Figure 5-5   Using CT to map out the x-ray density of structures and areas in the head. *(Thanks to Dr. Ray Carmody.)*

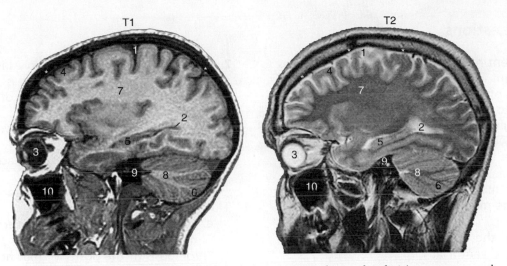

Figure 5-6   Using MRI to map out the distribution of water (and protons in other molecules) in structures and areas in the head. In T1-weighted images, areas with a lot of water, such as subarachnoid CSF (*1*), ventricular CSF (*2*), and the vitreous of the eye (*3*) are dark; in T2-weighted images they are bright. In T1-weighted images, gray matter such as cerebral cortex (*4*), the hippocampus (*5*), and cerebellar cortex (*6*) is darker than white matter such as the deep white matter of the cerebrum (*7*) and cerebellum (*8*); in T2-weighted images, gray matter is lighter than white matter. In both kinds of images, areas with few protons, such as the inner table of the skull (*), the temporal bone (*9*), and the maxillary sinus (*10*) produce little signal and are dark. (*Thanks to Drs. Elena Plante and Ray Carmody.*)

with different appearances (Fig. 5-6), but areas with few protons, such as bone and air-filled cavities, give off little signal.

Disruption of CSF Circulation Can Cause Hydrocephalus

There are bottlenecks in the path of CSF circulation, both inside and outside the ventricular system. If circulation is obstructed, CSF production continues unabated and **hydrocephalus** results. If the obstruction cuts off the communication between some part of the ventricular system and subarachnoid space, the hydrocephalus is termed **noncommunicating**. If all parts of the ventricular system still communicate with at least some portion of subarachnoid space, the hydrocephalus is termed **communicating**. Noncommunicating hydrocephalus could be caused by processes that occluded an interventricular foramen, the aqueduct, or all three apertures of the fourth ventricle. Communicating hydrocephalus could be caused by obstruction of the tentorial notch (because CSF must pass through the notch on its way from the posterior fossa to the superior sagittal sinus) or the arachnoid villi; it could also be caused, at least theoretically, by overproduction of CSF.

Study Questions

1. A patient had a small tumor that obstructed the right interventricular foramen. Which part(s) of the ventricular system would be likely to expand as a result of this tumor?

2. The lightest areas in conventional CT scans are areas with the most
   a. air.
   b. bone.
   c. gray matter.
   d. white matter.
   e. water.

3. Parts of the thalamus border on the
   a. lateral ventricle.
   b. third ventricle.
   c. fourth ventricle.
   d. both (a) and (b).
   e. all of the above.

4. The median aperture is
   a. the channel through which a lateral ventricle communicates with the third ventricle.
   b. the channel in the midbrain through which the third and fourth ventricles communicate.
   c. an opening in the roof of the third ventricle near the pineal gland.
   d. an opening in the roof of the fourth ventricle in the mid-medulla.
   e. another term for the central canal of the spinal cord.

5. Choroid plexus is found in all of the following locations except the
   a. anterior horn of the lateral ventricle.
   b. body of the lateral ventricle.
   c. roof of the third ventricle.
   d. roof of the fourth ventricle.

6. A lipid-insoluble dye injected into an artery supplying choroid plexus would
   a. not be able to leak out of the choroidal capillaries.
   b. leak across the choroid plexus, but be stopped by the ependymal lining of the ventricle.
   c. leak out of the choroidal capillaries, but be stopped by the choroid epithelium.
   d. none of the above.

7. The principal mechanism involved in the formation of cerebrospinal fluid is
   a. ultrafiltration across the walls of choroidal capillaries.
   b. ultrafiltration across the pial layer of choroid plexus.
   c. active transport of substances across the walls of choroidal capillaries.
   d. active transport of substances across the choroid epithelium.
   e. active transport of substances across the walls of arachnoid villi.

8. Thrombosis of the posterior (but not the anterior) part of the superior sagittal sinus can cause increased intracranial pressure; some even claim it can produce hydrocephalus. Why?

9. The ___ should be dark in both T1- and T2-weighted MRI scans.
   a. cerebral cortex
   b. corpus callosum
   c. lateral ventricle
   d. petrous temporal bone
   e. subarachnoid space

10. Noncommunicating hydrocephalus could be caused by
    a. obstruction of the tentorial notch.
    b. obstruction of all three apertures of the fourth ventricle.
    c. obstruction of the cerebral aqueduct.
    d. any of the above.
    e. b or c.

Blood Supply of the Brain

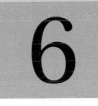

Chapter Outline

The central nervous system is tremendously active metabolically—relative to its weight, it uses much more than its share of the available oxygen and glucose. Corresponding to this metabolic activity, it has an abundant and closely regulated arterial supply and a large venous drainage system. Also, the CNS depends for its proper functioning on carefully controlled extracellular ion concentrations. Part of the basis for this control is a system of diffusion barriers, of which cerebral blood vessels are a major part.

The Internal Carotid Arteries and Vertebral Arteries Supply the Brain

Two interconnected arterial systems provide the blood supply to the brain (Fig. 6-1). The **internal carotid** system of each side supplies the ipsilateral cerebral

hemisphere, except for the medial surface of the occipital lobe and the medial and inferior surfaces of the temporal lobe. The **vertebral-basilar** system supplies those parts of the occipital and temporal lobes, as well as the brainstem and cerebellum. The supply of the diencephalon is shared by the two systems, with the vertebral/basilar system supplying most of the thalamus and the internal carotid system supplying most of the hypothalamus.

The Internal Carotid Arteries Supply Most of the Cerebrum

> **Key Concept**
>
> Small perforating arteries supply deep cerebral structures.

The internal carotid has two major terminal branches, the **anterior** and **middle cerebral arteries**. These are two of the three arteries that supply the cerebral cortex. On their way to their cortical areas of supply, both give rise to lots of small **perforating** or **ganglionic arteries** that supply most of the hypothalamus, basal ganglia, and internal capsule. (A comparable set from the vertebral-basilar system supplies the thalamus and brainstem.) The anterior and middle cerebral arteries have large terminal areas of distribution that are suggested to some extent by the name of each artery (Fig. 6-2).

The Vertebral-Basilar System Supplies the Brainstem and Parts of the Cerebrum and Spinal Cord

The two **vertebral arteries** fuse near the pontomedullary junction to form the single **basilar artery**, which ascends to the midbrain and terminates by bifurcating into the two **posterior cerebral arteries**. As they move along the brainstem, the vertebral and basilar arteries give off a series of branches; each has a name suggesting its terminal area of distribution (e.g., the **superior cerebellar artery** supplies the superior surface of the cerebellum). Along the way, each of these arteries provides perforating branches that supply the part of the brainstem it passes over. So knowing the levels at which these vertebral-basilar branches emerge (Fig. 6-3) provides a first approximation of the supply of the brainstem.

The Circle of Willis Interconnects the Internal Carotid and Vertebral-Basilar Systems

The internal carotid and vertebral/basilar systems are interconnected by a **posterior communicating artery**

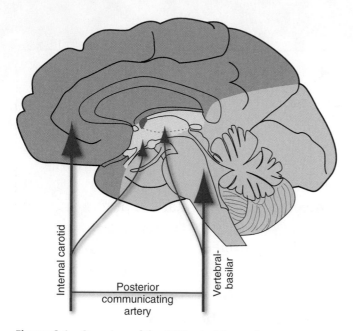

Figure 6-1 Overview of the CNS arterial supply.

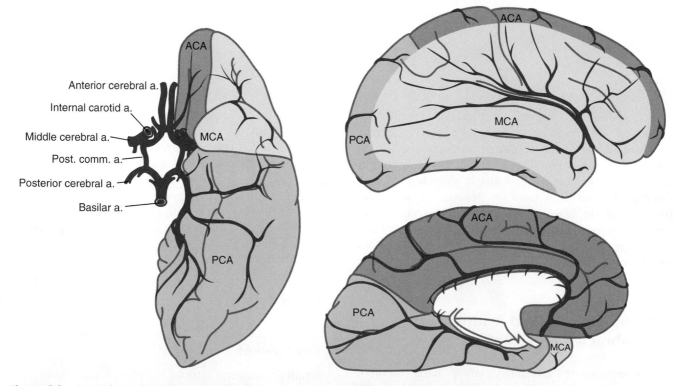

Figure 6-2 Arterial supply of the cerebral cortex. *ACA*, *MCA*, and *PCA* indicate areas supplied by the anterior, middle, and posterior cerebral arteries. *(Modified from Mettler FA: Neuroanatomy, ed 2. St. Louis, Mosby, 1948.)*

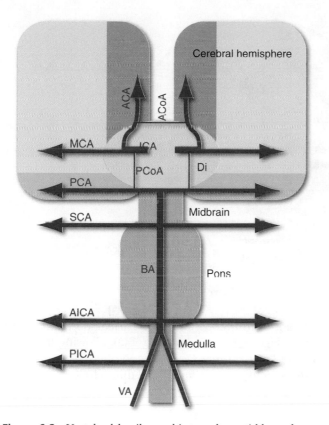

Figure 6-3 Vertebral-basilar and internal carotid branches. *ACA*, Anterior cerebral artery; *ACoA*, anterior communicating artery; *AICA*, anterior inferior cerebellar artery; *BA*, basilar artery; *Di*, diencephalon; *ICA*, internal carotid artery; *PCA*, posterior cerebral artery; *PCoA*, posterior communicating artery; *PICA*, posterior inferior cerebellar artery; *SCA*, superior cerebellar artery; *VA*, vertebral artery.

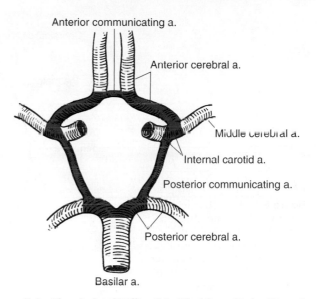

Figure 6-4 The circle of Willis. *(Modified from Hodes PJ et al: Am J Roentgenol 70:61, 1953.)*

Blood Flow to the CNS Is Closely Controlled

> ### Key Concept
>
> The overall flow rate is constant, but there are regional changes in blood flow.

on each side. In addition, the two anterior cerebral arteries are interconnected by the **anterior communicating artery**. These communicating arteries complete the arterial **circle of Willis** (Fig. 6-4). The communicating arteries are ordinarily fairly small and not capable of carrying much blood. However, in cases of slowly developing occlusions within the circle or in arteries leading into the circle, they can enlarge and provide a major alternative pathway for blood flow.

The numerous perforating or ganglionic arteries that leave the major arteries at the base of the brain (THB6 Figures 6-6 and 6-8, pp. 128 and 129)—many from within the circle of Willis, some from outside it—have an importance out of proportion to their size, because they supply deep structures where parts of multiple systems are packed together—places like the brainstem, diencephalon, and internal capsule. Damage to the internal capsule, for example, can disable major inputs to and outputs from a large expanse of cerebral cortex.

The total blood flow to the CNS, unlike that to most other organs, stays nearly constant no matter how you use your brain. Flow is maintained during changes in blood pressure by a process of **autoregulation**. If blood pressure drops, cerebral arterioles dilate; this compensates for the loss of pressure and lets the same amount of blood through. Conversely, if blood pressure rises, cerebral arterioles constrict.

Even though total flow to the brain remains constant, more of this flow goes to areas of the brain that are active at any given moment (THB6 Box 6-2, pp. 135-137). This is a local response to changes in extracellular metabolites and neurotransmitter release, mediated in large part by astrocytes. There is also autonomic innervation of cerebral vessels, but the physiological significance of this innervation is not clear.

Imaging Techniques Allow Arteries and Veins To Be Visualized

Increasing the contrast between blood and brain by any of several methods makes it possible to produce images of cerebral arteries and veins. Injecting radiopaque dyes makes blood vessels stand out when the head is examined with x-rays (THB6 Figures 6-15 and 6-16, pp. 133 and 134). Alternatively, MRI can also pick up flowing

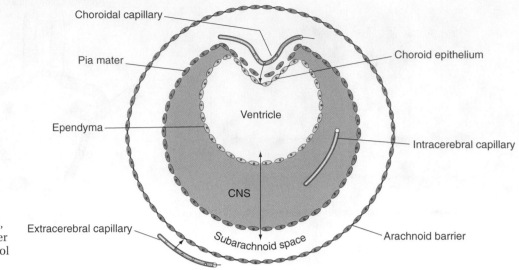

Figure 6-5 Brain barrier system. Solutes can diffuse freely through CSF-filled spaces and between neurons, but components of the barrier system (in blue letters) control what gets into these spaces.

blood, even without the injection of contrast agents (THB6 Figure 6-17, p. 134).

Strokes Result from Disruption of the Vascular Supply

Disruption of the arterial supply to an area of CNS for more than a few minutes (i.e., a **stroke**), either from hemorrhage or from occlusion of an artery, causes damage that is largely irreversible. Because the major CNS arteries have consistent distributions, strokes involving particular arteries produce distinctive signs and symptoms. For example, primary visual cortex is in the medial part of the occipital lobe, which is supplied by the posterior cerebral artery, so occlusion of this artery causes visual field deficits. Similarly, occlusion of a middle cerebral artery causes weakness and somatosensory deficits on the contralateral side.

A System of Barriers Partially Separates the Nervous System from the Rest of the Body

The **arachnoid barrier layer** (see Chapter 4) prevents things from diffusing into subarachnoid space from outside the CNS. The **choroid epithelium** (see Chapter 5) regulates what gets into newly formed cerebrospinal fluid. The last part of the barrier system between the CNS and the rest of the body is an array of tight junctions between the endothelial cells of CNS capillaries. This **blood-brain barrier** prevents substances from diffusing out of CNS capillaries and allows the endothelial cells to regulate what gets into CNS extracellular space. Collectively these three barriers (Fig. 6-5) make up a system that separates the extracellular spaces of the CNS from the general extracellular spaces of the body. A few small sites in the walls of the

third and fourth ventricles don't have a blood-brain barrier (THB6 Figures 6-29 and 6-30, p. 143), allowing these **circumventricular organs** to either monitor the composition of the systemic circulation or add things to it.

Superficial and Deep Veins Drain the Brain

> ### Key Concepts
>
> Most superficial veins empty into the superior sagittal sinus.
> Deep veins ultimately empty into the straight sinus.

Two sets of veins cooperate in the drainage of the brain (Figs. 6-6 and 6-7). **Superficial veins**, as their name

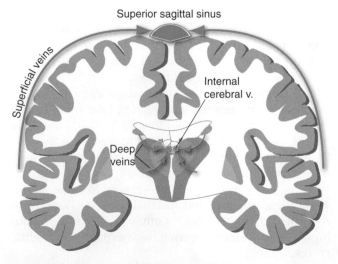

Figure 6-6 Overview of CNS venous drainage.

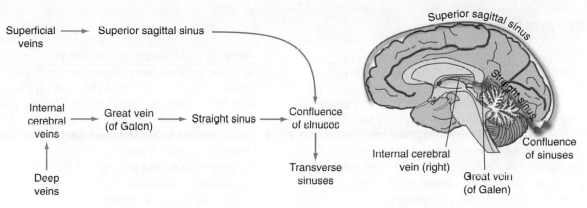

Figure 6-7 Arrangement and interconnections of superficial and deep veins.

implies, lie on the surface of each cerebral hemisphere and mostly drain upward or backward into the **superior sagittal sinus** (THB6 Figure 6-33, p. 145). **Deep veins**, in contrast, mostly drain structures in the walls of the ventricles and converge on the **internal cerebral veins** above the roof of the third ventricle (THB6 Figures 6-34 and 6-35, p. 146).

The two internal cerebral veins join to form the **great cerebral vein** (**of Galen**), which then joins the **straight sinus**. The superficial and deep drainage systems meet at the **confluence of the sinuses**, where the superior sagittal and straight sinuses join each other. From here, blood flows into the **transverse sinuses** and then reaches the **sigmoid sinuses** and the **internal jugular veins**.

Study Questions

1. A 62-year-old, right-handed lizard trainer, while berating a badly behaving basilisk, had the sudden onset of a headache and weakness of his left arm and leg. He looked in a mirror and noted that the left side of his face had begun to droop. He complained that the left side of his body felt "numb," and he was found to have diminished touch and position sense on the left. His visual fields were intact, and his cranial nerve examination was completely normal. An hour later his symptoms had resolved completely. The most likely cause of this transient deficit was temporary occlusion of the
   a. left anterior cerebral artery.
   b. right anterior cerebral artery.
   c. left middle cerebral artery.
   d. right middle cerebral artery.
   e. left posterior cerebral artery.
   f. right posterior cerebral artery.
   g. left vertebral artery.
   h. right vertebral artery.

2. The caudal pons receives much of its blood supply from the
   a. vertebral artery.
   b. posterior inferior cerebellar artery.
   c. anterior inferior cerebellar artery.
   d. superior cerebellar artery.
   e. posterior cerebral artery.

3. The cingulate gyrus receives most of its arterial supply from branches of the
   a. anterior cerebral artery.
   b. middle cerebral artery.
   c. posterior cerebral artery.
   d. superior cerebellar artery.
   e. vertebral artery.

4. Which of the following receive most of their blood supply from the middle cerebral artery? If any do not, which other artery is involved in each instance?
   a. superior frontal gyrus
   b. gyrus rectus
   c. superior temporal gyrus
   d. inferior temporal gyrus
   e. midbrain
   f. postcentral gyrus
   g. precentral gyrus
   h. medial surface of the occipital lobe

5. What clinical symptoms would you expect from a blood clot midway along the right posterior communicating artery? What would happen if the left posterior communicating artery became occluded sometime later?

6. The circle of Willis includes parts of all the following *except* the
   a. internal carotid artery.
   b. posterior cerebral artery.
   c. middle cerebral artery.
   d. anterior cerebral artery.
   e. posterior communicating artery.

7. The parahippocampal gyrus receives most of its arterial supply from branches of the
   a. anterior cerebral artery.
   b. internal carotid artery.
   c. middle cerebral artery.
   d. posterior cerebral artery.
   e. superior cerebellar artery.

8. An erythrocyte traveling from a distal branch of the middle cerebral artery to the internal jugular vein would traverse all of the following *except* the
   a. superior sagittal sinus.
   b. internal cerebral vein.
   c. confluence of the sinuses.
   d. transverse sinus.

9. Sites where small protein molecules would meet a major diffusion barrier include
   a. capillaries in the choroid plexus.
   b. the pia mater over the surface of the brain.
   c. a layer of cells in the arachnoid.
   d. all of the above.
   e. none of the above.

10. A 39-year-old handball hustler sat down in the corner of the court to take a break after beating 17 consecutive opponents. He started to watch a handball rolling across the court. A budding neurologist in the stands told a companion that the total blood flow to the handball hustler's brain didn't change much when he started watching the ball; instead, it increased in some areas (e.g., visual areas) and decreased in others. Was this correct?
    a. Yes
    b. No

Electrical Signaling by Neurons

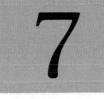

Chapter Outline

A Lipid/Protein Membrane Separates Intracellular and Extracellular Fluids

The Resting Membrane Potential of Typical Neurons Is Heavily Influenced, but Not Completely Determined, by the Potassium Concentration Gradient

Concentration Gradients Are Maintained by Membrane Proteins That Pump Ions

Inputs to Neurons Cause Slow, Local Potential Changes

Membrane Capacitance and Resistance Determine the Speed and Extent of the Response to a Current Pulse

Action Potentials Convey Information over Long Distances

Opening and Closing of Voltage-Gated Sodium and Potassium Channels Underlies the Action Potential

Action Potentials Are Followed by Brief Refractory Periods

Action Potentials Are Propagated without Decrement along Axons

---

Neurons share many properties with other cells, including their complement of organelles, an electrical potential across their surface membranes, and an ability to secrete various substances. What distinguishes neurons is the ways in which they have adapted these common properties for their roles as information-processing and information-conveying devices. For example, neurons have specialized configurations of organelles to support their extended anatomy (see Chapter 1). Similarly, they have adapted secretory processes to communicate with each other rapidly and precisely (see Chapter 8), and individual neurons use alterations in their **membrane potentials** to convey information between their various parts (this chapter).

This chapter provides an introductory explanation of how (1) membrane potentials develop and are maintained; (2) neurons use relatively **slow potential changes** (**graded potentials**) for computational purposes and to convey information over short distances; and (3) neurons use larger, briefer **action potentials** to convey information over longer distances.

A Lipid/Protein Membrane Separates Intracellular and Extracellular Fluids

Key Concepts

The lipid component of the membrane is a diffusion barrier.

Membrane proteins regulate the movement of solutes across the membrane.

Ions diffuse across the membrane through ion channels—protein molecules with pores.

The number and selectivity of ion channels determines the membrane potential.

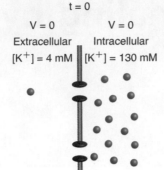

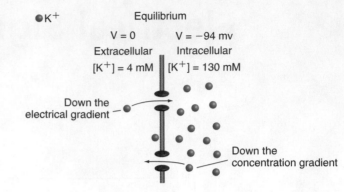

Figure 7-1 Production of a membrane potential by K⁺ channels and a K⁺ concentration gradient. Very few ions need to move in order to create this potential, so there is no significant change in K⁺ concentration on either side of the membrane.

The surface membrane of neurons, like that of other cells, is a double layer of lipid molecules with proteins embedded in it. Just as oil and water don't mix very well, the lipid part of the membrane is impermeable to water-soluble substances, prominently including the ions whose movement is central to electrical signaling. Subsets of the proteins embedded in the lipid bilayer are specialized to allow or even facilitate the movement of ions across the membrane. Some are hollow **ion channels** with a central, aqueous pore whose size and charged lining determines which kinds of ions can pass through; others are **ion pumps** that use metabolic energy to move specific ions across the membrane.

Changes in membrane potential over periods of milliseconds are produced by changes in current flow across the membrane. This is accomplished by changes in the conformation of some ion channels. Most or all channels can switch back and forth between states in which ions can pass through them easily ("open") and states in which they cannot ("closed"). Some channels can be induced to spend more time in one state or the other by changes in membrane potential (**voltage-gated channels**), others by the binding of some chemical, or ligand (**ligand-gated channels**).

The Resting Membrane Potential of Typical Neurons Is Heavily Influenced, but Not Completely Determined, by the Potassium Concentration Gradient

The K⁺ concentration inside neurons is much higher than that outside (because of ion pumps described a little later), and their surface membranes contain numerous **K⁺ channels** that are usually in the open state. If these were the only ion channels in the membrane, the following scenario would develop. The **concentration gradient** would drive K⁺ ions outward through the channels, creating a deficit of positive charges inside the cell. Opposite charges attract each other, so after a very small number of K⁺ ions had left, the resulting intracellular negativity would pull K⁺ ions back into the cell. At some point the concentration gradient and the **electrical gra-**

dient would exactly counterbalance each other, and K⁺ ions would enter and leave at equal rates (Fig. 7-1). The system would be in **equilibrium**, with no net movement of K⁺ in either direction and no energy requirement to stay that way. The transmembrane potential at which this occurs, the **potassium equilibrium potential** or V_K, is a logarithmic function of the concentration gradient and is specified by the **Nernst equation** (THB6 Appendix 7B, p. 176). At body temperature, a tenfold change in the K⁺ concentration on one side of the membrane causes a 62 mv change in V_K.

In reality, however, the K⁺ channels are not 100% selective for K⁺, and not all the channels in a resting membrane are K⁺ channels. As a result, Na⁺ ions are also able to flow across the membrane. The Na⁺ concentration outside neurons is much higher than that inside, so Na⁺ moves into the cell because of both the concentration gradient and the intracellular negativity. The result is competing ion flows (Fig. 7-2)—inward Na⁺ flow trying to move the membrane potential to V_{Na} and outward K⁺ flow trying to move the membrane potential to V_K—and a **steady state** is reached at a potential somewhere between V_{Na} and V_K. Just where the steady state is reached is determined by which ion the membrane is more permeable to (THB6 Appendix 7B, p. 176). Hence, V_{Na} and V_K are **boundary values** for the membrane potential, and changes in membrane **permeability** to Na⁺ or K⁺ will cause the membrane potential to move closer to one or the other; this is the usual basis for electrical signaling by neurons. The membranes of most neurons most of the time are much more permeable to K⁺ than to Na⁺, so the resting membrane potential is close to V_K.

Concentration Gradients Are Maintained by Membrane Proteins That Pump Ions

A major difference between the theoretical K⁺-selective membrane and the real-life membrane permeable to both K⁺ and Na⁺ is that energy is required to maintain the concentration gradients across real-life membranes. If K⁺ continually flowed out and Na⁺ continually flowed

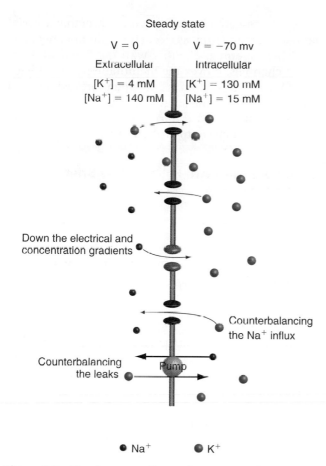

Steady state

V = 0   V = −70 mv

Extracellular   Intracellular

$[K^+]$ = 4 mM $[K^+]$ = 130 mM
$[Na^+]$ = 140 mM $[Na^+]$ = 15 mM

Down the electrical and
concentration gradients

Counterbalancing
the Na^+ influx

Counterbalancing
the leaks   Pump

● Na^+ ● K^+

Figure 7-2 Development of a steady-state membrane
potential.

in, the ionic concentration gradients across the membrane would fade away and the membrane potential would decline toward zero. This is averted by another class of membrane-spanning proteins, ion pumps, that use the energy liberated by hydrolysis of ATP to pump ions in the opposite direction and so maintain concentration gradients. The best known example is the **Na^+/ K^+ exchange pump** that pumps Na^+ out and K^+ in, compensating for the steady-state leakage through channels.

Inputs to Neurons Cause Slow, Local Potential Changes

Inputs to neurons, whether at **synapses** (see Chapter 8) or in the receptive portion of **sensory receptors** (see Chapter 9), cause ion channels to open or close for milliseconds or longer. As a result, current flow through the channels increases or decreases and the membrane potential at the input site moves toward V_{Na} (**depolarization**) or V_K (**hyperpolarization**). The current flows and voltage changes spread passively through nearby parts

of the neuron in a way that depends on the electrical properties of those parts.

Membrane Capacitance and Resistance Determine the Speed and Extent of the Response to a Current Pulse

Key Concepts

Membranes have a time constant, allowing temporal summation.
Larger diameter neuronal processes have longer length constants.

Biological membranes behave electrically like combinations of **capacitors** (the lipid bilayer) and **resistors** (the ion channels). The gory details are recounted in THB6 Appendix 7A (p. 173), but suffice it to say for these purposes that capacitor/resistor combinations change the time course of electrical signals, slowing them down and smearing them out in time. So abruptly opening and then closing an ion channel causes not a square-wave voltage change, but rather one that builds up exponentially when the channel opens and then decays exponentially when the channel closes. Although this seems initially like a terrible way to build a signaling system, it actually has computational advantages, because it allows neurons to sum up multiple signals that are not quite simultaneous (**temporal summation**; see THB6 Figure 7-7, p. 157). The rate at which voltage changes (the **time constant**) determines the degree of temporal summation.

Current entering a neuron at one point spreads in all available directions, and before long all of it leaks out, either by passing through other ion channels or by changing the charge on the membrane capacitance. How far it spreads (i.e., the **length constant**) depends on things like the diameter of the neuronal process in question. Current takes the path of least resistance in its travels and, all other factors being equal, it is easier for current to move longitudinally through a large-diameter process than to squeeze through ion channels. Hence large-diameter dendrites and axons have long length constants and small-diameter ones have short length constants. This passive spread allows **spatial summation** of graded neuronal input signals arising at slightly different sites (THB6 Figure 7-9, p. 159).

Action Potentials Convey Information over Long Distances

Length constants are not very long, and graded electrical signals spreading passively in even the largest axons and dendrites would die out in a few millimeters. Neurons commonly need to convey messages over distances equal to hundreds or thousands of length constants and use **action potentials** (also called **spikes** or **nerve impulses**) to do so. Action potentials are fundamentally different from graded **postsynaptic potentials** and **receptor potentials** in several ways: They are large, brief, and always depolarizing; have a **threshold;** and are **propagated** actively along axons rather than dying out.

Opening and Closing of Voltage-Gated Sodium and Potassium Channels Underlies the Action Potential

Action potentials are produced by the coordinated activity of special **voltage-gated Na+ channels** and **K+ channels** (Fig. 7-3), and areas of membrane that have sufficient quantities of these channels are electrically excitable (i.e., are able to produce action potentials). Depolarization of such an area of membrane (e.g., by depolarizing current flow from a nearby synapse) causes the voltage-gated Na+ channels to begin opening, which depolarizes the membrane even more. If enough channels are opened by the initial depolarization (i.e., the depolarization reaches threshold), this Na+ channel opening builds on itself explosively until most of the channels are open, Na+ permeability is greater than K+ permeability, and the membrane potential moves close to V_{Na}. This depolarization is short-lived, however, because the Na+ channels spontaneously enter a closed, **inactivated** state and cannot reopen until they are "reset" (**deinactivated**) by having the membrane potential return to near the resting level.

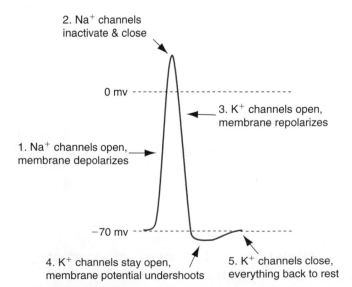

1. Na+ channels open, membrane depolarizes

2. Na+ channels inactivate & close

3. K+ channels open, membrane repolarizes

4. K+ channels stay open, membrane potential undershoots

5. K+ channels close, everything back to rest

Figure 7-3 Production of an action potential by the coordinated opening and closing of voltage-gated Na+ channels and K+ channels.

The voltage-gated K+ channels are slower than the Na+ channels, opening only as the action potential nears its peak. Their opening, together with the inactivation of the Na+ channels, moves the membrane potential back toward V_K. The K+ channels stay open for a while even after all the Na+ channels have closed, causing an after-hyperpolarization phase during which the membrane potential is even closer to V_K than usual.

Action Potentials Are Followed by Brief Refractory Periods

> **Key Concept**
>
> Refractory periods limit the repetition rate of action potentials.

The inactivation of voltage-gated Na+ channels has important consequences for the production of subsequent action potentials. For a brief period after the peak of an action potential, so many channels are inactivated that another action potential cannot be generated. This is the **absolute refractory period**, which grades into a **relatively refractory period** during which less than the full complement of channels is available. As a result, threshold is elevated because a greater percentage of this reduced population must be activated in order to produce another action potential. Because an action potential and the absolute refractory period following it last a millisecond or two, the maximum firing rate of neurons is about 1 kHz. The relative refractory period ensures that even this upper limit is rarely reached.

Action Potentials Are Propagated without Decrement along Axons

> **Key Concepts**
>
> Refractory periods ensure that action potentials are propagated in only one direction.
> Propagation is continuous and relatively slow in unmyelinated axons.
> Action potentials jump rapidly from node to node in myelinated axons.

Neurons typically have a **trigger zone** with a low threshold, near where the axon emerges from the cell body, where action potentials are initiated (Fig. 7-4). Inputs to the dendrites and cell body sum temporally and spatially, spread passively (**electrotonically**) to the trigger zone, and initiate one or more action potentials

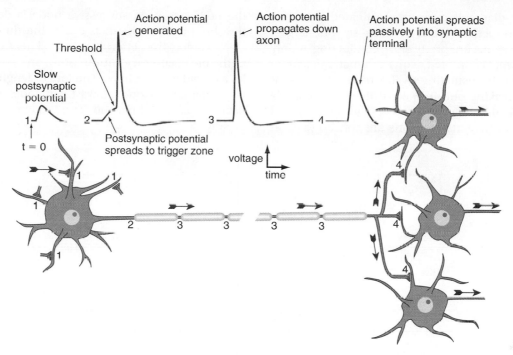

Figure 7-4   Overview of electrical signaling by neurons.

if threshold is reached. Once initiated, an action potential spreads passively both down the axon and back into the cell body (THB6 Figure 7-13, p. 162). Cell bodies usually lack sufficient numbers of voltage-gated Na⁺ channels to make action potentials, so that's the end of the story in that direction. The axon, on the other hand, has lots of them, so spread of the action potential in that direction brings neighboring regions to threshold and the action potential propagates down the axon. Once the action potential reaches the end of the axon, it cannot

turn around and propagate back toward the cell body because the regions just traversed are refractory.

Unmyelinated axons have voltage-gated Na⁺ channels distributed all along them, and the action potential spreads down these axons by having each successive area of membrane depolarize to threshold (Fig. 7-5). It takes time for the channels to open, so the conduction velocity of action potentials in unmyelinated axons is limited by how far down the axon a depolarizing current spreads (i.e., by the length constant of the axon). Hence,

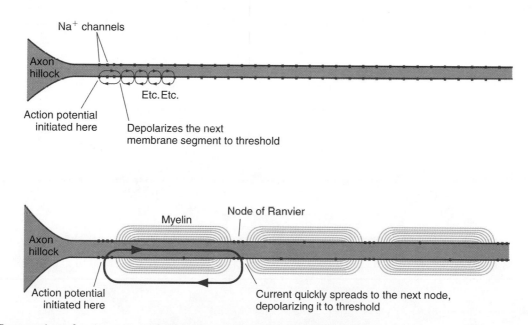

Figure 7-5   Propagation of action potentials along unmyelinated and myelinated axons.

the larger the diameter of an unmyelinated axon, the faster the **conduction velocity**. Even so, our largest unmyelinated axons are pretty slow, conducting at only about 2.5 m/sec. **Myelinated axons** conduct much more rapidly because the insulating myelin internodes prevent current from leaking out. Instead, it flows very rapidly from one **node of Ranvier** to the next. The voltage-gated Na^+ channels of myelinated axons are concentrated at the nodes, so each successive node is depolarized to threshold and its channels open (the time-consuming step). Hence, the action potential skips from one node to the next (**saltatory conduction**), and conduction can be as rapid as 100 m/sec. The longer length constant of large-diameter axons allows their nodes to be spaced farther apart, so here too larger axons conduct more rapidly.

Study Questions

For questions 1-5, use the following list of possibilities:

    a. Depolarization.
    b. Hyperpolarization.
    c. No change.

What would be the effect of each of the following on the membrane potential of a typical neuron?

1. Closing K^+ channels.
2. Closing Na^+ channels.
3. Increasing the extracellular Na^+ concentration.
4. Decreasing the extracellular K^+ concentration.
5. Application for several hours of a drug that blocked the Na^+/K^+ exchange pump.

6. A dendrite with which of the following combinations of properties would have the longest length constant?
    a. Large diameter, few open channels.
    b. Large diameter, many open channels.
    c. Small diameter, few open channels.
    d. Small diameter, many open channels.

For questions 7-9, match the listed experimental treatments with the expected changes in action potential waveform.

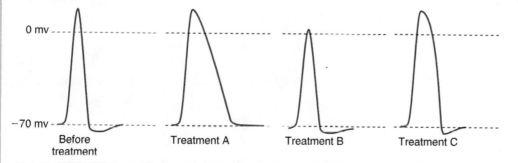

0 mv

−70 mv

Before treatment   Treatment A   Treatment B   Treatment C

7. Decreasing the extracellular Na^+ concentration.
8. Applying a drug that prevents the opening of voltage-gated K^+ channels.
9. Applying a drug that slows the inactivation of voltage-gated Na^+ channels.

10. Which of the following axons would be expected to have the fastest conduction velocity?
    a. 0.5 μm diameter, myelinated.
    b. 0.5 μm diameter, unmyelinated.
    c. 1.5 μm diameter, myelinated.
    d. 1.5 μm diameter, unmyelinated.

Synaptic Transmission between Neurons

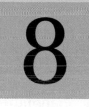

In contrast to the way in which information travels *within* individual neurons as electrical signals, information is usually transmitted *between* neurons through the release of **neurotransmitters** at specialized junctions called **synapses**. And in contrast to unvarying, always depolarizing action potentials, a wide variety of slow **graded potentials** may be produced at the synapses on an individual neuron—some depolarizing, some hyperpolarizing, some milliseconds in duration, others seconds, minutes, or even hours.

There Are Five Steps in Conventional Chemical Synaptic Transmission

The fundamental elements of a chemical synapse (Fig. 8-1) are a **presynaptic ending** from which neurotransmitter is released, a **synaptic cleft** across which it diffuses, and a **postsynaptic element** containing **receptor molecules** to which the neurotransmitter binds. Although the presynaptic ending is usually an axon terminal and the postsynaptic ending usually a dendrite, any part of a neuron can be presynaptic to any part of another neuron. The essential processes at chemical synapses are presynaptic **synthesis**, **packaging**, and **release** of neurotransmitter; binding to postsynaptic **receptors**; and **termination** of neurotransmitter action.

Neurotransmitters Are Synthesized in Presynaptic Endings and in Neuronal Cell Bodies

As described a little later, most neurotransmitters are either **small molecules** (e.g., amino acids) or **peptides**. Small-molecule transmitters are synthesized in presynaptic cytoplasm by soluble enzymes that arrived there by slow axonal transport. Peptide transmitters are synthesized in the cell body, loaded into vesicles, and shipped to presynaptic endings by fast axonal transport.

Neurotransmitters Are Packaged into Synaptic Vesicles before Release

Neurotransmitters are packaged for release from presynaptic endings in collections of **synaptic vesicles** (THB6 Figure 8-5, p. 181). All presynaptic endings contain a complement of **small vesicles**, with specific transporters in their walls that pack them full of small-molecule transmitters. Many also contain some less numerous **large vesicles** containing peptides shipped from the cell body; one or more small-molecule transmitters are often added to the brew in these large vesicles. Small vesicles are located near the presynaptic membrane, whereas large vesicles are usually located farther away.

Presynaptic Endings Release Neurotransmitters into the Synaptic Cleft

Neurotransmitter release is a secretory process triggered by an increase in presynaptic Ca^{2+} concentration. The membranes of presynaptic terminals contain **voltage-gated Ca^{2+} channels** that open when an action potential spreads into the terminal (Fig. 8-2). Ca^{2+} influx causes one or more vesicles to fuse with the presynaptic membrane and dump its neurotransmitter content into the synaptic cleft. Because small vesicles are close to the synaptic cleft, they are the first to release their contents. Because the large vesicles are farther away, release of

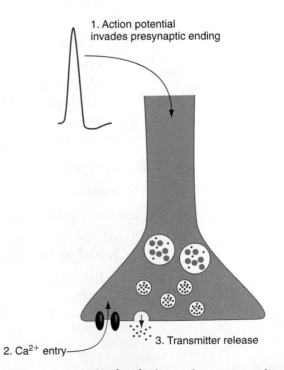

1. Action potential invades presynaptic ending

2. Ca^{2+} entry

3. Transmitter release

Figure 8-2 Calcium-stimulated release of neurotransmitter.

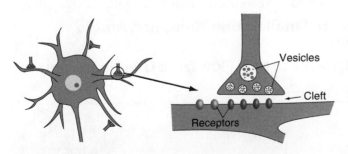

Vesicles

Cleft

Receptors

Figure 8-1 Cartoon of a typical chemical synapse.

their contents requires more Ca^{2+} entry (hence, more presynaptic action potentials) and more time.

Neurotransmitters Diffuse Across the Synaptic Cleft and Bind to Postsynaptic Receptors

The effects of neurotransmitters are mediated by receptors situated in or near postsynaptic membranes. Receptors for the transmitters in small vesicles are mostly located right across the synaptic cleft, contributing to the rapid action of these transmitters. Receptors for peptides are often located outside the synaptic cleft, contributing to the slowness of large-vesicle effects.

Neurotransmitter Action Is Terminated by Uptake, Degradation, or Diffusion

A concerted effort is made to remove neurotransmitter soon after it is released so that the postsynaptic element will be prepared for subsequent releases. Several different mechanisms are used, with different kinds of synapses emphasizing different mechanisms. Most commonly, transmitter is taken back up by the presynaptic ending or by nearby glial cells, but some transmitters are degraded by enzymes in the synaptic cleft or simply diffuse away.

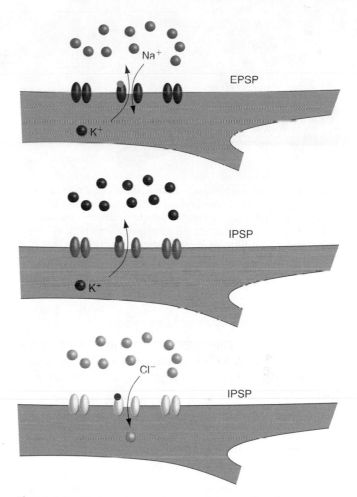

Figure 8-3   Fast postsynaptic potentials, mediated by binding of small-molecule transmitters to ligand-gated ion channels.

Synaptic Transmission Can Be Rapid and Point-to-Point, or Slow and Often Diffuse

Postsynaptic responses to transmitter binding can be either depolarizing or hyperpolarizing. Because depolarizing and hyperpolarizing events move the postsynaptic membrane closer to or farther from threshold, they are referred to respectively as **excitatory postsynaptic potentials (EPSPs)** and **inhibitory postsynaptic potentials (IPSPs)**. Depending on the synapse and the transmitter, both EPSPs and IPSPs can be either fast (lasting a few milliseconds) or slow.

Rapid Synaptic Transmission Involves Transmitter-Gated Ion Channels

Fast EPSPs and IPSPs are produced by the binding of neurotransmitter to a receptor that is itself a **ligand-gated ion channel** (Fig. 8-3); because of the direct coupling to ion flow, these are also referred to as **ionotropic** receptors. The permeability change induced by the binding of transmitter determines the postsynaptic response. Some receptors become permeable to both Na$^+$ and K$^+$, causing depolarization (EPSP). Others

become permeable to K$^+$ or Cl$^-$, causing hyperpolarization (IPSP).

Slow Synaptic Transmission Usually Involves Postsynaptic Receptors Linked to G Proteins

Slow EPSPs and IPSPs are produced by a multistep process involving changes in the postsynaptic concentration of a **second messenger**. They typically begin with binding of neurotransmitter to a receptor linked to an adjacent **guanine nucleotide-binding protein (G protein)**. The G protein then dissociates and one of its subunits triggers subsequent steps. In the simplest case, the G protein subunit is itself the second messenger and binds to a ligand-gated ion channel (Fig. 8-4). In most cases, however, the G protein subunit increases or decreases the activity of an enzyme, which in turn causes

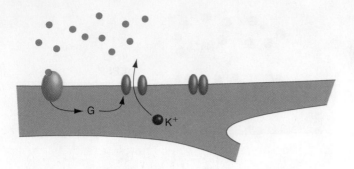

Figure 8-4 Slow postsynaptic potentials, usually mediated by binding of small-molecule transmitters or peptides to G protein-coupled receptors and subsequent dissociation of G proteins. G protein subunits (G) can have a variety of effects. They can be as simple as the indicated opening of a channel but are usually more complex, involving activation of an enzyme or even alteration of gene expression.

changes in the concentration of something else. Because of the intermediate metabolic steps, the receptors involved in slow EPSPs and IPSPs are also referred to as **metabotropic** receptors.

The Postsynaptic Receptor Determines the Effect of a Neurotransmitter

Although some neurotransmitters usually have either excitatory or inhibitory effects, the nature of the postsynaptic response to a transmitter is actually determined by the postsynaptic receptor. Hence, a given neurotransmitter can produce EPSPs at some synapses and IPSPs at others, or slow postsynaptic potentials at some synapses and fast ones at others. For example, acetylcholine, the first neurotransmitter discovered, produces fast EPSPs at neuromuscular junctions (by binding to **nicotinic receptors** there) and slow EPSPs or IPSPs at other synapses (by binding to **muscarinic receptors**).

The Size and Location of a Synaptic Ending Influences the Magnitude of Its Effects

All chemical synapses have the basic elements just described, but nevertheless come in a variety of configurations with different functional characteristics. Most CNS presynaptic endings, for example, are tiny, contain vesicles clustered for release at just one or a few **active zones**, and produce very small postsynaptic potentials in response to a presynaptic action potential. Neuromuscular endings and a few specialized CNS presynaptic endings, in contrast, contain many active zones and produce large postsynaptic potentials in response to a presynaptic action potential (THB6 Figure 8-13, p. 187). The proximity of a synapse to the trigger zone for action potential production also has important implications for the effects of transmitter release. Postsynaptic potentials initiated far out on a dendrite will largely die out as they spread passively toward the trigger zone, whereas those initiated near the trigger zone will reach it with little decrement.

Presynaptic Endings Can Themselves Be Postsynaptic

The synapses mentioned so far have effects on the entire postsynaptic neuron, increasing or decreasing the likelihood that it will fire. Another, more selective, kind of synapse is one in which a presynaptic terminal receives synaptic inputs from other axon terminals, suppressing or facilitating Ca^{2+} entry into the terminal. The resulting **presynaptic inhibition** or **presynaptic facilitation** is a clever mechanism for selectively affecting only selected outputs from one neuron to another (THB6 Figure 8-15, p. 188).

Synaptic Strength Can Be Facilitated or Depressed

The amount of transmitter released by a presynaptic terminal in response to an action potential invading it is not constant, but rather depends on the history of activity in that terminal. There are several short-lived processes that result in the release of more or fewer vesicles (**potentiation** and **depression**, respectively). Other processes lasting for days or longer involve insertion or removal of postsynaptic receptors. The resulting **long-term potentiation** or **long-term depression** is thought to play a fundamental role in learning and memory.

Messages Also Travel Across Synapses in a Retrograde Direction

The synaptic transmission described so far is the mechanism used to convert electrical activity in one neuron into electrical activity in other neurons. However, there is also chemical signaling in the opposite direction that is electrically silent and does not depend on synaptic vesicles. Membrane-derived **endocannabinoids**, gases such as **nitric oxide** and **carbon monoxide**, and larger molecules that serve as **growth factors** can all be released by postsynaptic neurons and have effects on presynaptic endings or neurons.

Most Neurotransmitters Are Small Amine Molecules, Amino Acids, or Neuropeptides

Key Concepts

Acetylcholine mediates rapid, point-to-point transmission in the PNS.

Amino acids mediate rapid, point-to-point transmission in the CNS.

Amines and neuropeptides mediate slow, diffuse transmission.

Nearly all neurotransmitters are either small molecules (**amines** or **amino acids**) or **neuropeptides**. There are dozens of known or suspected neuropeptide transmitters, but a much smaller number of important **small-molecule transmitters**, each with a more or less distinctive role (Tables 8-1 and 8-2). **Acetylcholine** mediates rapid, point-to-point, excitatory transmission in the PNS. **Glutamate** and γ-**aminobutyric acid (GABA)** mediate rapid excitatory and inhibitory transmission, respectively, in the CNS. Amines and neuropeptides almost without exception mediate slow, second-messenger effects in the CNS and PNS.

Gap Junctions Mediate Direct Current Flow from One Neuron to Another

A minority of synaptic connections eschews neurotransmitters altogether, and instead are **gap junctions** at which current can flow directly from one neuron into another (Fig. 8-5). These electrical synapses are useful for groups of neurons that need to fire synchronously and for networks of neurons designed to spread information laterally with little computation, but otherwise are fairly rare in the mammalian CNS.

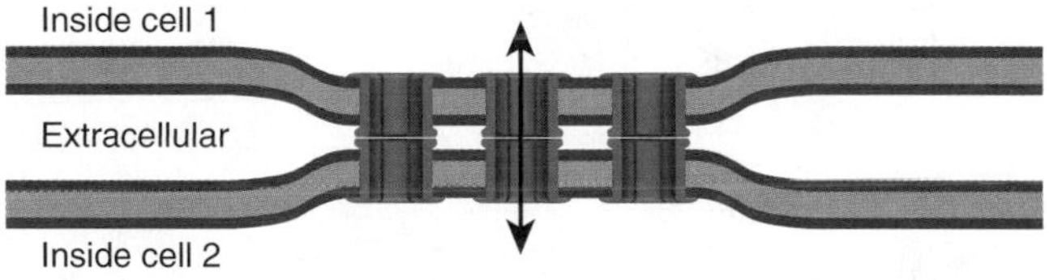

Table 8-1	Principal small-molecule transmitters

Amines
  Acetylcholine
  Monoamines
    Serotonin
    Catecholamines
      Dopamine
      Norepinephrine

Amino acids
  Glutamate
  GABA (γ-aminobutyric acid)

Figure 8-5   A gap junction, the substrate of electrical synapses.

Table 8-2 Structures, locations, and actions of the principal small-molecule transmitters

Transmitter	Principal Neurons Using It	Major Action*
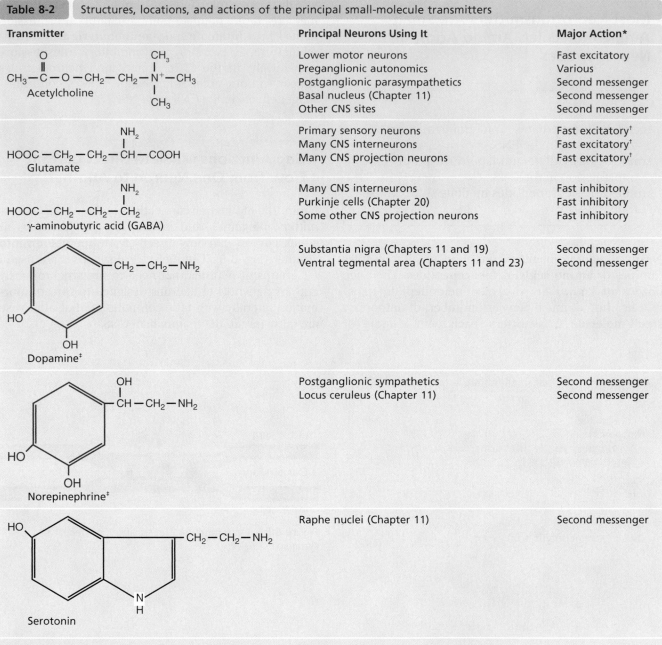 Acetylcholine	Lower motor neurons Preganglionic autonomics Postganglionic parasympathetics Basal nucleus (Chapter 11) Other CNS sites	Fast excitatory Various Second messenger Second messenger Second messenger
Glutamate	Primary sensory neurons Many CNS interneurons Many CNS projection neurons	Fast excitatory[†] Fast excitatory[†] Fast excitatory[†]
γ-aminobutyric acid (GABA)	Many CNS interneurons Purkinje cells (Chapter 20) Some other CNS projection neurons	Fast inhibitory Fast inhibitory Fast inhibitory
Dopamine[‡]	Substantia nigra (Chapters 11 and 19) Ventral tegmental area (Chapters 11 and 23)	Second messenger Second messenger
Norepinephrine[‡]	Postganglionic sympathetics Locus ceruleus (Chapter 11)	Second messenger Second messenger
Serotonin	Raphe nuclei (Chapter 11)	Second messenger

*Major but not all actions. For example, there are metabotropic glutamate and GABA receptors.
[†]Important exception: the NMDA receptor (THB6 Figure 8-20, p. 193) has additional voltage-gated properties.
[‡]The blue part is the catechol group for which catecholamines are named.

Study Questions

1. Monoamine neurotransmitters include all of the following *except*
   a. acetylcholine.
   b. dopamine.
   c. norepinephrine.
   d. serotonin.

2. Neuropeptides and small-molecule transmitters are *both* synthesized to a great extent in
   a. neuronal cell bodies.
   b. presynaptic endings.
   c. both a and b.
   d. None of the above is correct.

Answer questions 3-9 using the following list. Each item may be used once, more than once, or not at all.

   a. Acetylcholine.
   b. Dopamine.
   c. Norepinephrine.
   d. Serotonin.
   e. Glutamate.
   f. GABA.

3. Released by motor neurons at neuromuscular junctions.

4. A transmitter used by Purkinje cells, which convey the inhibitory output from cerebellar cortex.

5. Released by preganglionic autonomic neurons.

6. The principal excitatory transmitter in the CNS.

7. Released by small inhibitory interneurons in the cerebral cortex.

8. A neurotransmitter with second-messenger effects released by neurons of the substantia nigra.

9. Released by the central endings of primary sensory neurons.

10. Stimulation of motor cortex causes action potentials in corticospinal axons and EPSPs in the motor neurons they terminate on. The basis of these EPSPs is typically the opening of
    a. ligand-gated Cl^- channels.
    b. ligand-gated K^+ channels.
    c. ligand-gated Na^+/K^+ channels.
    d. voltage-gated Cl^- channels.
    e. voltage-gated K^+ channels.
    f. voltage-gated Na^+/K^+ channels.

Sensory Receptors and the Peripheral Nervous System

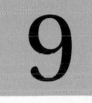

Chapter Outline

Receptors Encode the Nature, Location, Intensity, and Duration of Stimuli

Each Sensory Receptor Has an Adequate Stimulus, Allowing It to Encode the Nature of a Stimulus

Many Sensory Receptors Have a Receptive Field, Allowing Them to Encode the Location of a Stimulus

Receptor Potentials Encode the Intensity and Duration of Stimuli

Most Sensory Receptors Adapt to Maintained Stimuli, Some More Rapidly Than Others

Sensory Receptors All Share Some Organizational Features

Sensory Receptors Use Ionotropic and Metabotropic Mechanisms to Produce Receptor Potentials

All Sensory Receptors Produce Receptor Potentials, but Some Do Not Produce Action Potentials

Somatosensory Receptors Detect Mechanical, Chemical, or Thermal Changes

Nociceptors Have Both Afferent and Efferent Functions

Receptors in Muscles and Joints Detect Muscle Status and Limb Position

Visceral Structures Contain a Variety of Receptive Endings

Peripheral Nerves Convey Information to and from the CNS

The Diameter of a Nerve Fiber Is Correlated with Its Function

---

Neural traffic to and from the CNS travels in **peripheral nerves**. The afferent fibers in these peripheral nerves either have endings that respond to physical stimuli (making them **primary afferents** that are also **sensory receptors**) or carry information from separate sensory receptor cells in the periphery. The efferent fibers end on muscle fibers, autonomic ganglia, or glands.

Receptors Encode the Nature, Location, Intensity, and Duration of Stimuli

The job of sensory receptors collectively is to produce electrical signals that represent all relevant aspects of stimuli—what kind of stimulus, where it is, how intense, when it starts and stops. Sometimes a single receptor can do all of this, but often one or more populations of receptors are required.

Each Sensory Receptor Has an Adequate Stimulus, Allowing It to Encode the Nature of a Stimulus

Sensory receptors **transduce** ("lead across") some aspect of the external or internal environment into a graded electrical signal (a **receptor potential**). Each receptor is more sensitive to one kind of stimulus, called its **adequate stimulus**, than to others. Hence, there are **chemoreceptors**, **photoreceptors**, **thermoreceptors**, and **mechanoreceptors**, and the identity of the particular receptors responding to a stimulus provides some initial information about the nature of that stimulus. Individual types of receptors within these broad classes are usually more finely tuned to particular aspects of a stimulus category, providing even more information about the nature of a stimulus. For example, although all the mechanoreceptors of the inner ear are very similar to each other, some are set up to respond best to sound vibrations, others to the position of the head (see Chapter 14).

Many Sensory Receptors Have a Receptive Field, Allowing Them to Encode the Locations of a Stimulus

Some receptors are tuned not only to their adequate stimulus, but also to the location of the stimulus. All receptors obviously can only respond to stimuli that reach them, but some receptors and their central connections are specialized to preserve information about location. For example, single cutaneous receptors respond only to stimuli that affect areas of skin containing their endings, and the CNS keeps track of which individual receptors respond in order to determine the location of a touch or pinch. An area of the body or outside world in which stimuli cause electrical changes in a receptor is called the **receptive field** of that receptor and, because this spatial information is preserved in sensory pathways, neurons located more centrally in these pathways also have receptive fields.

For some other receptors, receptive fields either are less relevant or the concept just doesn't apply. Examples are many **visceral receptors** keeping track of things like blood pressure or glucose concentration, or vestibular receptors monitoring head position.

Receptor Potentials Encode the Intensity and Duration of Stimuli

To a first approximation, receptors encode the intensity and duration of stimuli by the size and duration of the receptor potentials they produce (Fig. 9-1). There's actu-

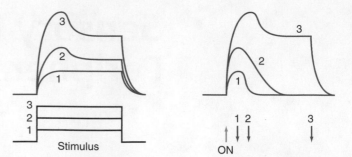

Figure 9-1 Coding of the intensity (*left*) and duration (*right*) of stimuli by the receptor potentials of a generic sensory receptor. As is the case in most receptors, the response adapts (declines) during intense or prolonged stimuli.

ally a little more to it than this, though, because in some systems increasing intensity is signaled by recruiting additional, less sensitive, receptors (e.g., rods for dim light and cones for bright light). In addition, some receptors signal only the beginning and end of a stimulus and do not respond to maintained stimuli.

Most Sensory Receptors Adapt to Maintained Stimuli, Some More Rapidly Than Others

Some receptors produce a maintained response to a constant stimulus, and so are called **slowly adapting**. The response of others declines and may disappear entirely during a constant stimulus; these are called **rapidly adapting**. Rapidly adapting receptors can therefore act like miniature differentiators, producing a constant response to a steadily changing stimulus. The classic example of a rapidly adapting receptor is the **Pacinian corpuscle** (THB6 Figure 9-8, p. 209), which responds only briefly at the beginning and end of a constant mechanical stimulus, but responds continuously to vibration.

Most receptors, unlike the two shown in Fig. 9-2, are actually somewhere between the extremes of slowly and rapidly adapting. The response may be exaggerated at the beginning (or end) of a stimulus, but maintained to some extent throughout the stimulus (see Fig. 9-1).

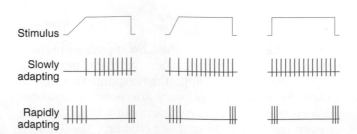
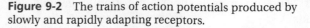

Figure 9-2 The trains of action potentials produced by slowly and rapidly adapting receptors.

Sensory Receptors All Share Some Organizational Features

Sensory receptors, like neurons in general, have parts specialized for receiving stimuli (in this case sensory rather than synaptic stimuli) and parts specialized for transmitting information to other neurons (THB6 Figure 9-4, p. 205). They also typically have numerous mitochondria near the receptive area, presumably to supply energy for transduction processes.

Sensory Receptors Use Ionotropic and Metabotropic Mechanisms to Produce Receptor Potentials

The transduction mechanisms used by sensory receptors are gratifyingly similar to the mechanisms used in the production of postsynaptic potentials (Fig. 9-3). Some are depolarizing, others hyperpolarizing; some

Table 9-1	Transduction mechanisms used by different kinds of sensory receptors	
Stimulus-Gated Channels	**G Protein–Coupled Mechanisms**
Most somatosensory receptors	Some pain receptors Photoreceptors
Hair cells (CN VIII)	Olfactory receptors
Some taste receptors	Some taste receptors
Some visceral receptors	Some visceral receptors

use direct alteration of ion channels, others use G protein coupled mechanisms (Table 9-1). Many of the receptor molecules used by sensory receptors are actually closely related to postsynaptic receptor molecules, but are simply set up so that they respond to a stimulus rather than to a neurotransmitter.

All Sensory Receptors Produce Receptor Potentials, but Some Do Not Produce Action Potentials

Receptor potentials are not propagated actively; rather, like postsynaptic potentials, they decay over a short distance. Therefore, receptors that signal over long distances must generate action potentials as well as receptor potentials (Fig. 9-4). An example is a receptor that signals something touching your big toe. It produces a depolarizing receptor potential in response to touch, but the receptor potential itself dies out near the receptive ending. But action potentials are initiated at a nearby trigger zone and get conducted all the way into the CNS. In mammals, receptors with long axons convey information about **somatic sensation** (touch, pain, etc.), **visceral sensation,** and **smell,** and all produce depolarizing receptor potentials.

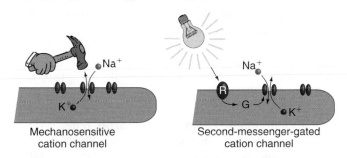

Mechanosensitive cation channel   Second-messenger-gated cation channel

Figure 9-3   The two general kinds of transduction mechanisms. Channels directly sensitive to stimuli are typified by the directly mechanosensitive channels found in a wide variety of receptors, including those sensitive to touch, sound, and osmolality. The example of a G protein–coupled mechanism shown here is a retinal photoreceptor (a rod), in which the photopigment (rhodopsin, *R*) is closely related to a postsynaptic norepinephrine receptor; however, other receptors, such as olfactory receptors, also use G protein–coupled mechanisms.

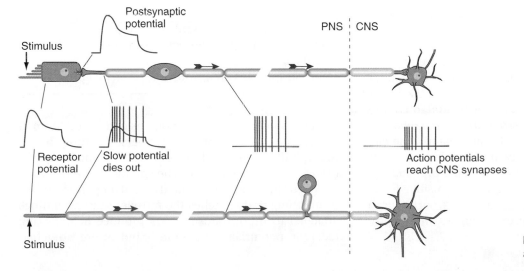

Figure 9-4   Receptors with and without long axons.

In contrast, receptors that signal over short distances (less than a mm or so) don't need to produce action potentials. Instead, they synapse on the peripheral processes of primary afferent neurons, whose cell bodies lie in peripheral ganglia. The receptor potential changes the rate at which the receptor releases transmitter, and this in turn changes the rate at which the primary afferent sends action potentials into the CNS. A receptor with a short axon or no axon can depolarize (and release more transmitter) or hyperpolarize (and release less transmitter) in response to a stimulus; some can do both, depending on the specifics of the stimulus. Examples of short receptors are **taste receptor cells**, **photoreceptors**, and the mechanoreceptive **hair cells** of the inner ear.

Somatosensory Receptors Detect Mechanical, Chemical, or Thermal Changes

Key Concepts

Cutaneous receptors have either encapsulated or nonencapsulated endings.
Capsules and accessory structures influence response properties of cutaneous mechanoreceptors.
Nociceptors, thermoreceptors, and some mechanoreceptors have free nerve endings.
Cutaneous receptors are not distributed uniformly.

Somatosensory receptors have peripheral processes that end in places like skin, muscle, or joints and have long axons, cell bodies in dorsal root ganglia (or cranial nerve ganglia), and central processes that end in the CNS. Some of the peripheral processes, particularly those of pain and temperature receptors, are simply **free nerve endings**. Others have **encapsulated endings** and/or various types of **accessory structures** (two such muscle receptors are described a little later). The capsules and accessory structures play a role in coupling stimuli to receptive endings; the capsule of a Pacinian corpuscle, for example, is largely responsible for its being rapidly adapting. Capsules also have barrier properties that can regulate the environment of receptive endings.

Receptive endings are not distributed uniformly, but instead are more densely packed in areas where fine acuity or control is needed. For example, the fingertips have many receptive endings per unit area, which begins to account for the detailed tactile discriminations we can perform using our fingertips (THB6 Figure 9-9, p. 210, and see Box 9-1, p. 210, for another striking example).

Nociceptors Have Both Afferent and Efferent Functions

Pain receptors (**nociceptors**) are different in some respects from other receptors, in ways that fit with our common experiences with tissue-damaging stimuli. Injured parts of the body become extra sensitive to painful stimuli (**hyperalgesia**) and can hurt even in response to a usually innocuous stimulus (**allodynia**), both partially the result of pain-sensitive endings becoming more sensitive (rather than adapting, like most other receptors would). In addition, the skin surrounding an injured area becomes red and swollen (edematous) as a result of signals traveling peripherally over other branches of the same pain receptors that signal the injury: When afferent action potentials reach a branch point they can propagate not only centrally, but also peripherally through an **axon reflex** (THB6 Figure 9-13, p. 214). (This is the only known reflex involving only one neuron and no part of the CNS.) Depolarization reaching nociceptive endings causes peripheral release of neurotransmitters, which in turn causes redness and swelling.

Receptors in Muscles and Joints Detect Muscle Status and Limb Position

Key Concepts

Muscle spindles detect muscle length.
Golgi tendon organs detect muscle tension.
Joints have receptors.
Muscle spindles are important proprioceptors.

Muscle spindles are receptor organs composed of small muscle fibers (called **intrafusal fibers**, meaning "inside the spindle") enclosed in a spindle-shaped capsule (THB6 Figure 9-14, p. 216). The spindles are embedded in skeletal muscles and oriented so that they are stretched by anything that stretches the muscle. Sensory endings attached to the intrafusal fibers produce depolarizing receptor potentials when the spindles are stretched

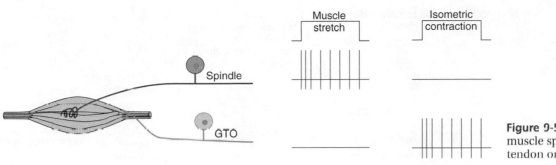

Figure 9-5 Responses of muscle spindles and Golgi tendon organs (GTO).

(Fig. 9-5). The ends of intrafusal fibers are contractile and receive inputs from small (**gamma**) motor neurons. Contraction of this part of an intrafusal fiber does not contribute significantly to the strength of a muscle. Rather, it regulates the length of the central, stretch-sensitive portion of the intrafusal fiber and thereby regulates its sensitivity to externally applied stretch (THB6 Figure 9-15, p. 217).

Golgi tendon organs are networks of sensory endings interspersed among the collagen fibers of tendons (THB6 Figure 9-16, p. 218). Tension in a tendon compresses the sensory endings and causes depolarizing receptor potentials. Passive muscle stretch does not generate much tension in a tendon, but muscle contraction against a load does (see Fig. 9-5).

Joints also contain a variety of mechanosensitive endings. These were thought for a time to be critically important for position sense (**proprioception**), but it is now known that at most joints, muscle spindles and sometimes cutaneous receptors are more important.

Visceral Structures Contain a Variety of Receptive Endings

Visceral structures also receive a wealth of receptive endings, but much less is known about them than about somatosensory and other receptors. Collectively they form the afferent components of a vast network of connections mediating the homeostatic and drive-related behaviors discussed in Chapter 23.

Peripheral Nerves Convey Information to and from the CNS

Key Concept

Extensions of the meninges envelop peripheral nerves.

The dura mater surrounding the CNS continues as the **epineurium** of peripheral nerves (Fig. 9-6; see THB6 Figure 9-19, p. 222). This is a substantial covering around each nerve, conferring considerable mechanical strength. The arachnoid continues as the **perineurium** covering individual nerve fascicles. Just as in the case of the arachnoid, perineurial cells are interconnected by tight junctions and form a diffusion barrier between the inside and the outside of a nerve fascicle, part of a continuation of the blood-brain barrier system as a **blood-nerve barrier** (capillaries inside nerve fascicles are zipped up by tight junctions, helping to complete the barrier). The **endoneurium** is the loose background connective tissue within nerve fascicles.

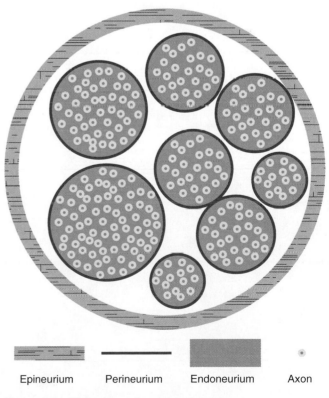

| Epineurium | Perineurium | Endoneurium | Axon |

Figure 9-6 Wrappings of peripheral nerves.

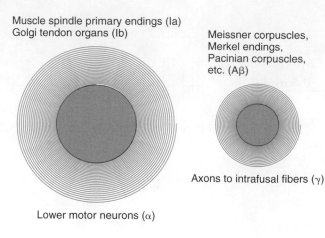
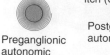

Figure 9-7 Relative sizes of peripheral nerve axons and their myelin sheaths, and the functions associated with different sizes. Some of the jargon used to describe fibers of different sizes is indicated in parentheses.

The Diameter of a Nerve Fiber Is Correlated with Its Function

Large-diameter axons have large cell bodies and thick myelin sheaths, and they conduct action potentials rapidly. Small-diameter axons have smaller cell bodies, have thin myelin sheaths or are unmyelinated, and conduct action potentials slowly. Large-diameter sensory axons end peripherally in muscle spindles, Golgi tendon organs, and joint receptors. The sensory axons that end peripherally as the cutaneous receptors used for discriminative tactile sense (precise judgments of shape and position) are not quite as large. Small-diameter axons end peripherally as receptors for pain, temperature, simple sensation of touch, and assorted visceral receptors. Major categories of somatic afferent fibers in peripheral nerves, and their relative sizes, are indicated in Fig. 9-7 (see THB6 Table 9-3, p. 224, for more details).

Efferent axons of different diameters are also associated with different functions. The largest myelinated axons innervate ordinary skeletal muscle. Those that innervate the intrafusal fibers of muscle spindles are smaller, and preganglionic autonomic fibers are smaller still. Postganglionic autonomic fibers are unmyelinated.

Study Questions

1. The term "adequate stimulus" refers to
   a. any stimulus that causes a particular receptor to increase the rate at which it produces action potentials.
   b. any stimulus that causes a particular receptor to depolarize.
   c. any stimulus that elicits the largest possible response from a particular receptor.
   d. the kind of stimulus to which a particular receptor is most sensitive.

2. Receptors with long axons
   a. produce receptor potentials that are actively propagated to the central nervous system.
   b. produce receptor potentials that decay passively, but change the rate at which the receptor generates action potentials.
   c. in mammals, produce depolarizing receptor potentials and increased rates of action potentials.
   d. None of the above is true.
   e. Both b and c are true.

3. A receptor with these stimulus-response properties would be classified as

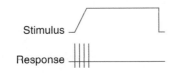

   a. slowly adapting.
   b. rapidly adapting.

4. Recordings from the axon of an unknown muscle receptor indicated that it fired more rapidly in response to muscle contraction, but did not respond much to passive stretch of the muscle. The receptor was most likely to be a
   a. muscle spindle.
   b. Golgi tendon organ.
   c. Pacinian corpuscle.
   d. None of these receptors has these response properties.

5. Selectively stimulating all the gamma motor neurons to a muscle would initially cause
   a. maximum contraction of the muscle.
   b. increased firing rates in all the afferent fibers from muscle spindles in that muscle.
   c. increased firing rates in all the afferents from Golgi tendon organs in that muscle.
   d. decreased firing rates in all the afferents from muscle spindles in that muscle.
   e. decreased firing rates in all the afferents from Golgi tendon organs in that muscle.

For questions 6-10, match the receptor types in the column on the left with the fiber characteristics in the column on the right. More than one fiber characteristic may apply to one receptor; indicate all that apply.

6. Afferents from Golgi tendon organs
7. Afferents from most touch receptors
8. Motor axons to ordinary skeletal muscle
9. Afferents from many pain receptors
10. Postganglionic autonomic axons

a. Large diameter
b. Small diameter
c. Heavily myelinated
d. Unmyelinated
e. None of the above

11. Most of the mechanical strength of peripheral nerves is a property of the
    a. axons themselves.
    b. endoneurium.
    c. epineurium.
    d. perineurium.

12. A diffusion barrier between the extracellular spaces inside and outside peripheral nerve fascicles is located in the
    a. endoneurium.
    b. epineurium.
    c. perineurium.

Spinal Cord

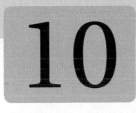

The spinal cord is pretty small, but it's important out of proportion to its size. It's the home of all the motor neurons that work your body, and of a large percentage of the autonomic motor neurons as well. It's also the recipient of nearly all the sensory information taken in by your body. Beyond that, many of the organizing principles of spinal cord reflexes and pathways apply to other parts of the CNS.

The Spinal Cord Is Segmented

Key Concept

The spinal cord is shorter than the vertebral canal.

Segments of the spinal cord (Fig. 10-1)—8 **cervical**, 12 **thoracic**, 5 **lumbar**, 5 **sacral**, 1 **coccygeal**—are defined by the spinal nerves formed from **dorsal** and **ventral roots** attached bilaterally to each segment. The spinal cord has a **cervical** and a **lumbar enlargement**, serving the needs of the arms and legs respectively, and ends at the pointed **conus medullaris**. The conus medullaris is located at vertebral level L1/L2, even though the dural sac surrounding the spinal cord extends to vertebral level S2. So dorsal and ventral roots from progressively more caudal levels need to travel progressively longer distances through spinal subarachnoid space before reaching their intervertebral foramina of entry or exit. The collection of spinal nerves in subarachnoid space caudal to the conus medullaris is the **cauda equina** (Latin for "horse's tail").

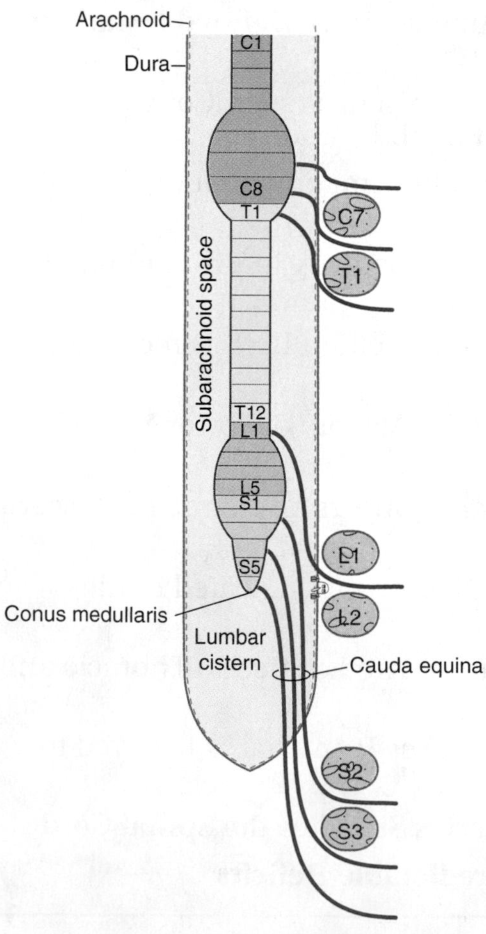

Spinal nerves C1-C7 use the foramen above the corresponding vertebra, C8 uses the foramen between vertebrae C7 and T1, and all others use the foramen below the corresponding vertebra.

Each Spinal Cord Segment Innervates a Dermatome

The mesoderm and ectoderm that develop adjacent to a given spinal cord segment go on to form bones, muscles, and skin in predictable locations. The resulting systematic relationships between cord segments and different muscles (THB6 Table 10-1, p. 231) and areas of skin (**dermatomes**; see THB6 Figure 10-4 and Table 10-2, pp. 231 and 232) are tremendously important in clinical neurology.

All Levels of the Spinal Cord Have a Similar Cross-Sectional Structure

The gray matter core of the spinal cord is roughly in the shape of an H with a dorsal-ventral orientation at all levels (Fig. 10-2). The dorsally directed limbs of the H are the **posterior** (or **dorsal**) **horns**, and the ventrally directed limbs are the **anterior** (or **ventral**) **horns**. The posterior horn, derived from the alar plate of the neural tube, is a sensory processing area that receives most of the afferents that arrive in ipsilateral dorsal roots. The anterior horn is derived from the basal plate and contains the motor neurons whose axons form the ventral roots. The **intermediate gray matter** between the anterior and posterior horns is a mixture of interneurons and tract cells in sensory and motor circuits; at some levels it also contains autonomic motor neurons with axons that leave in the ventral roots.

The anterior and posterior horns divide the surrounding spinal white matter into **anterior**, **lateral**, and **posterior funiculi** (funiculus is Latin for "string").

Figure 10-1 Overview of spinal cord gross anatomy.

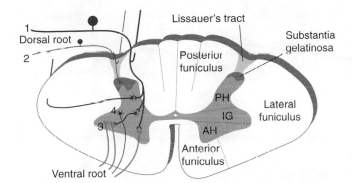

Figure 10-2 General cross-sectional anatomy of the spinal cord. At all levels, large-diameter (*1*) and small-diameter (*2*) sensory fibers enter through the dorsal root and feed into ascending pathways and reflex arcs; axons of lower motor neurons (*3*) leave through ventral roots. Some levels, as described a little later, also contain preganglionic autonomic neurons (*4*) with axons that leave through ventral roots. *AH*, Anterior horn; *IG*, intermediate gray; *PH*, posterior horn.

As dorsal roots approach the spinal cord, the afferent fibers sort themselves out so that large-diameter fibers enter medial to small-diameter fibers. The large-diameter fibers, carrying touch and position information, have some branches that travel rostrally in the posterior funiculus and others that end in deeper portions of the posterior horn. The small-diameter fibers, primarily carrying pain and temperature information, travel in the **dorsolateral fasciculus (Lissauer's tract)** to termination sites in a superficial zone of the posterior horn called the **substantia gelatinosa**.

The Spinal Cord Is Involved in Sensory Processing, Motor Outflow, and Reflexes

The wiring principles discussed in Chapter 3 are pretty apparent in the spinal cord. Central processes of primary afferents (cell bodies in **dorsal root ganglia**) are the only routes through which sensory information from the body can reach the spinal cord. They give rise to branches that feed into reflex circuits, into pathways to the thalamus, and into pathways to the cerebellum. These branches end in ipsilateral gray matter, mostly but not entirely in the posterior horn. **Lower motor neurons** in the anterior horn receive inputs from reflex circuits, as well as through descending pathways (i.e., axons of **upper motor neurons**), and project to ipsilateral muscles. They are the only routes through which the spinal cord can tell skeletal muscles to contract, and loss of lower motor neurons or their axons is followed by **flaccid paralysis** of the muscles they used to innervate—profound weakness, loss of tone and reflexes, and atrophy.

Spinal Gray Matter Is Regionally Specialized

Key Concepts

The posterior horn contains sensory interneurons and projection neurons.
The anterior horn contains motor neurons.
The intermediate gray matter contains autonomic neurons.

Some parts of the spinal gray matter (e.g., the substantia gelatinosa) are present in all segments. Others are either present at only some levels or emphasized at some levels in ways that make functional sense (THB6 Figure 10-8, p. 236). The most prominent examples of the former are **preganglionic sympathetic neurons**, present in the T1-L3 intermediate gray and forming a pointy **lateral horn** in thoracic segments; **preganglionic parasympathetic neurons**, present in the S2-S4 intermediate gray; and **Clarke's nucleus**, at the base of the posterior horn from T1-L2 and particularly prominent at lower thoracic levels. As an example of level-specific emphasis, an anterior horn is present at all levels but is enlarged laterally in the cervical and lumbar enlargements to accommodate all the lower motor neurons for distal muscles supplied by these levels.

Reflex Circuitry Is Built into the Spinal Cord

Key Concepts

Muscle stretch leads to excitation of motor neurons.
Painful stimuli elicit coordinated withdrawal reflexes.
Reflexes are accompanied by reciprocal and crossed effects.

Reflexes are involuntary, stereotyped responses to sensory inputs, and every kind of sensory input is involved in reflex circuitry of one or more types. The simplest kind of reflex imaginable (other than the axon reflex) involves a primary afferent and a lower motor neuron, with a synapse in the CNS connecting the two.

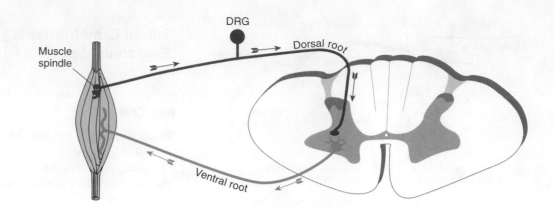

Figure 10-3 The stretch reflex arc.

This is the circuit underlying **stretch reflexes** (Fig. 10-3), through which a muscle contracts in response to being stretched. (Stretch reflexes are tested by tapping tendons and so they're often called **deep tendon reflexes**, even though the receptors that initiate them are located in muscle spindles and not tendons.)

Stretch reflexes are the only monosynaptic reflexes. All others involve one or more interneurons. An example is the **flexor reflex** (or **withdrawal reflex**), through which a limb is removed from a painful stimulus (Fig. 10-4). This reflex is considerably more complex than a stretch reflex because all the muscles of a limb, and therefore motor neurons in several spinal segments, come into play.

Reflexes are often depicted as isolated responses to a stimulus, but typically there are associated **reciprocal** and **crossed** effects that enhance their effectiveness. Tapping the patellar tendon stretches the quadriceps, which contracts in response; at the same time, hamstrings motor neurons are inhibited, making it easier for the quadriceps to shorten. As one foot is withdrawn from a painful stimulus, extensor motor neurons for the contralateral leg are automatically excited, making it easier for that leg to support the body.

Reflexes Are Modifiable

Despite the implication of the preceding description, reflex responses to a given stimulus in real-life situations actually vary from moment to moment. Part of the variation is produced by pathways descending from the brain to the spinal cord, regulating reflex sensitivity to suit different behavioral states. For example, think about how vigorously you might withdraw from something that touched you if you were vigilant and on edge in a scary situation, compared with the response to the same stimulus in a more relaxed setting. Part of the variation is built into movement patterns. For example, during some phases of walking, withdrawing from something that touches a foot would help avoid tripping or stumbling; during other phases, not withdrawing would help that leg bear weight.

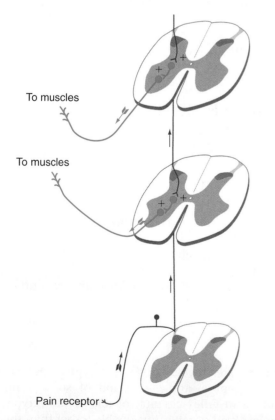

Figure 10-4 The flexor (withdrawal) reflex arc, which involves connections, through interneurons, in multiple spinal segments.

Ascending and Descending Pathways Have Defined Locations in the Spinal White Matter

There are only three pathways of major clinical significance in the spinal cord: the **posterior columns** (touch and position), **spinothalamic tract** (pain and temperature), and **lateral corticospinal tract** (commands for voluntary movements). Each has a consistent location at all cord levels (see Fig. 10-9 later in this chapter).

The Posterior Column–Medial Lemniscus System Conveys Information about Touch and Limb Position

Key Concepts

Information about the location and nature of a stimulus is preserved in the posterior column–medial lemniscus system.

Damage to the posterior column medial lemniscus system causes impairment of proprioception and discriminative tactile functions.

Large-diameter primary afferents, carrying touch and position information, have collaterals that ascend through the ipsilateral posterior funiculus. Incoming collaterals add on lateral to those already present in the posterior column, so by cervical levels each posterior column is subdivided into a medial **fasciculus gracilis**, representing the leg, and a more lateral **fasciculus cuneatus**, representing the arm (Fig. 10-5). Fasciculi gracilis and cuneatus then terminate in **nuclei gracilis** and **cuneatus**, the **posterior column nuclei** of the caudal medulla. Second order fibers from neurons of the posterior column nuclei cross the midline and form the **medial lemniscus**, which ascends through the brainstem to the thalamus (to a thalamic nucleus called the ventral posterolateral nucleus (VPL), for reasons explained in Chapter 16). VPL neurons then project to somatosensory cortex of the postcentral gyrus and adjacent areas.

There's a well-defined, modality-specific **somatotopic** organization at all levels of this pathway, which makes it easier to keep track of details about the nature and location of stimuli.

The Spinothalamic Tract Conveys Information about Pain and Temperature

Key Concept

Damage to the anterolateral system causes diminution of pain and temperature sensations.

The most important pathway for pain and temperature information is the spinothalamic tract (Fig. 10-6); it also carries some touch information. Spinothalamic

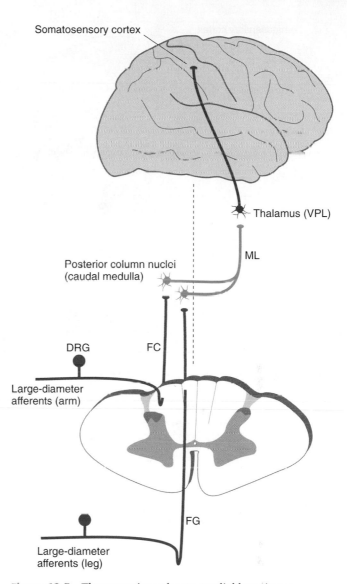

Figure 10-5 The posterior column–medial lemniscus pathway. *DRG,* Dorsal root ganglion; *FC,* fasciculus cuneatus; *FG,* fasciculus gracilis; *ML,* medial lemniscus.

neurons (i.e., the second order cells) are located in the posterior horn, so this pathway, unlike the posterior column-medial lemniscus pathway, crosses the midline in the spinal cord. Small-diameter primary afferents, carrying pain and temperature and some touch information, traverse Lissauer's tract and end on spinothalamic neurons in the posterior horn. Small interneurons of the substantia gelatinosa regulate the transmission of information at this synapse. The axons of spinothalamic neurons then cross the midline and form the spinothalamic tract, which ascends through the brainstem to VPL and to other thalamic nuclei as well (corresponding to pain usually having a more widespread effect on attention and mood than touch does). These thalamic neurons then project to somatosensory cortex of the postcentral

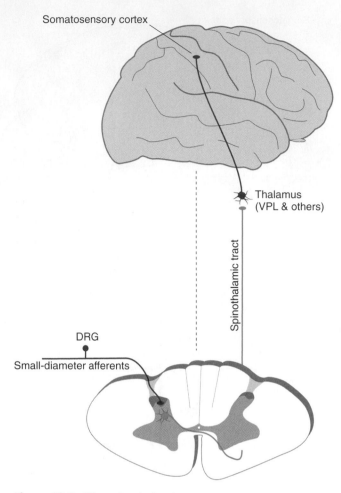

Figure 10-6 The spinothalamic tract.

gyrus and some other cortical areas (again, more widespread than touch information). Intermingled with these direct spinothalamic fibers are other axons that convey pain and temperature information from the posterior horn to the thalamus indirectly, by way of the reticular formation, and to other sites as well. The entire collection of ascending pain and temperature fibers is often referred to collectively as the **anterolateral pathway** because of its position in the spinal cord.

Additional Pathways Convey Somatosensory Information to the Thalamus

Most kinds of information travel in more than one pathway in the spinal cord and elsewhere, so damage to a single tract seldom causes total loss of a function. For example, some touch information travels through the spinothalamic tract, and some touch and position information travels in other tracts in the lateral funiculus. However, for each function there is usually one

pathway that is more important than all the others—the posterior column-medial lemniscus system for touch and position, the spinothalamic tract for pain and temperature.

Spinal Information Reaches the Cerebellum Both Directly and Indirectly

> **Key Concepts**
>
> The posterior spinocerebellar tract and cuneocerebellar tract convey proprioceptive information.
> The anterior spinocerebellar tract conveys more complex information about the leg.

One job of the cerebellum is to compare the movements actually being made to the movements the CNS thinks it is trying to make, and then issue correcting signals if there is a discrepancy. To do this, the cerebellum needs information from the spinal cord about the current position of limbs and other body parts. Some of it reaches the cerebellum indirectly, by way of the reticular formation and other brainstem sites, but there is also a group of spinocerebellar tracts that convey this information directly to the cerebellum (THB6 Figure 10-23, p. 250). The **anterior** and **posterior spinocerebellar tracts** convey information about the leg. The **cuneocerebellar tract** is just like the posterior spinocerebellar tract, except that it arises in the medulla from the **lateral cuneate nucleus** and conveys information about the arm.

Descending Pathways Influence the Activity of Lower Motor Neurons

> **Key Concept**
>
> The corticospinal tracts mediate voluntary movement.

The most important pathway for the control of voluntary movement is the **corticospinal tract** (also called the **pyramidal tract** because its fibers travel through the pyramids on the ventral surface of the medulla). Corticospinal neurons are located in the precentral gyrus and adjacent cortical areas. Their axons descend through the internal capsule (bypassing the thalamus) and travel in a ventral location in the brainstem, passing through the cerebral peduncle (on the ventral surface of the midbrain), the basal pons, and the medullary pyramids (Fig. 10-7). Most of these fibers then

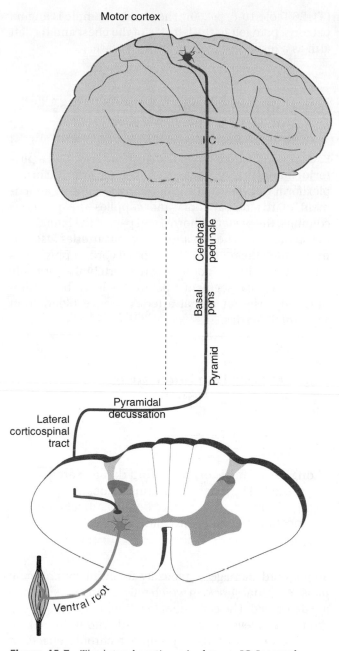

Figure 10-7 The lateral corticospinal tract. *IC*, Internal capsule.

cross the midline in the **pyramidal decussation** at the medulla-spinal cord junction and enter the lateral corticospinal tract. (The few uncrossed fibers enter the **anterior corticospinal tract** in the anterior funiculus.) Corticospinal fibers then end on motor neurons or interneurons of the spinal gray matter. Just as in the case of sensory pathways, there are additional, parallel routes for some of this input to reach the spinal cord, so destruction of the corticospinal tract causes weakness but not total paralysis. For example, projections from the vestibular nuclei of the brainstem to the spinal cord (vestibulospinal tracts) provide one alternate route.

Neurons that project to lower motor neurons are called **upper motor neurons**, and damage to them causes a distinctive type of weakness. Reflex circuitry survives and, over time, becomes more influential than normal; **hyperreflexia** and increased muscle tone result. In addition, some normally suppressed spinal circuitry is unmasked and several pathological reflexes emerge. The most famous of these is **Babinski's sign** (dorsiflexion of the big toe and fanning of the others in response to firmly stroking the sole of the foot).

The Autonomic Nervous System Monitors and Controls Visceral Activity

The **autonomic nervous system** (**ANS**) does not project efferents from the CNS directly to smooth or cardiac muscles or to glands. Instead, **preganglionic** autonomic neurons in the CNS project through the ventral roots to **postganglionic** neurons in ganglia outside the CNS (Fig. 10-8). These postganglionic neurons then project to target organs. (The only exception is the adrenal medulla, which receives autonomic (sympathetic) projections directly from the CNS.) Preganglionic axons are thinly myelinated, while postganglionic axons are unmyelinated.

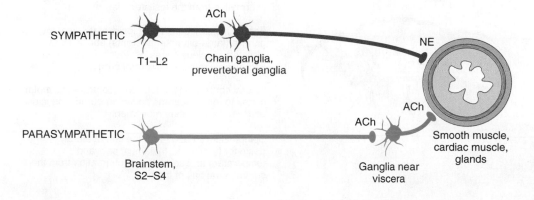

Figure 10-8 General layout of sympathetic and parasympathetic neurons. *ACh*, Acetylcholine; *NE*, norepinephrine.

Preganglionic Parasympathetic Neurons Are Located in the Brainstem and Sacral Spinal Cord

The **parasympathetic** subdivision of the ANS, in a very general sense the energy-absorption and energy-storage part of the system, has most of its preganglionic neurons in the brainstem, but some in the sacral spinal cord. The postganglionic neurons are located in ganglia near or in the target organs. Both preganglionic and postganglionic parasympathetic neurons use acetylcholine as a neurotransmitter.

Preganglionic Sympathetic Neurons Are Located in Thoracic and Lumbar Spinal Segments

The **sympathetic** subdivision of the ANS, in a very general sense the "fight or flight" part of the system, has all its preganglionic neurons in the intermediate gray matter of the thoracic and upper lumbar spinal cord (the **intermediolateral cell column**, forming a lateral horn). The postganglionic neurons are located relatively close to the spinal cord in **sympathetic chain ganglia** and **prevertebral ganglia**. Preganglionic sympathetic neurons, like preganglionic parasympathetics, use acetylcholine as a neurotransmitter. In contrast, almost all postganglionic sympathetic neurons use norepinephrine.

Visceral Distortion or Damage Causes Pain That Is Referred to Predictable Dermatomes

Spinal cord segments that contain preganglionic autonomic neurons also receive afferents from visceral structures. Most of the central endings of these afferents participate in things like autonomic reflexes and updating the brainstem and hypothalamus about visceral goings on. Some, however, synapse on the same spinothalamic tract neurons that signal somatic pain. The result is that visceral damage or distortion produces pain that is **referred** to some predictable somatic area, providing valuable clinical clues about disease processes (THB6 Table 10-8, p. 260). The classic example is angina pectoris, pain felt in the left side of the chest and the left arm as a result of coronary artery disease.

A Longitudinal Network of Arteries Supplies the Spinal Cord

Each vertebral artery gives rise to an **anterior** and a **posterior spinal artery**. The posterior spinal arteries form a plexiform network that travels along the line of attachment of the dorsal roots and supplies the posterior columns, the posterior horns, and part of the lateral corticospinal tract. The two anterior spinal arteries fuse and travel along the midline of the spinal cord, supplying its anterior two thirds. Blood from the vertebral artery only reaches cervical segments; below this level, both anterior and posterior spinal arteries receive blood from segmental arteries.

Spinal Cord Damage Causes Predictable Deficits

> **Key Concepts**
>
> Long-term effects of spinal cord damage are preceded by a period of spinal shock.
> The side and distribution of deficits reflects the location of spinal cord damage.

Spinal cord damage is typically followed by an acute phase of **spinal shock**, in which reflexes and muscle tone are depressed. The consistent locations of tracts and cell groups at all levels of the spinal cord (Fig. 10-9) make it possible to predict the subsequent chronic effects of

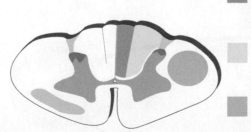

Figure 10-9 Summary of major spinal cord tracts, as seen at a lower cervical level. The spinothalamic and corticospinal tracts are present at all levels. Below about T6, the posterior column system is represented only by fasciculus gracilis.

Fasciculus gracilis. From ipsilateral dorsal root ganglia (large-diameter afferents) below T6 to ipsilateral nucleus gracilis; touch and position information from the ipsilateral leg.

Fasciculus cuneatus. From ipsilateral dorsal root ganglia (large-diameter afferents) above T6 to ipsilateral nucleus cuneatus; touch and position information from the ipsilateral arm.

Lateral corticospinal tract. From contralateral motor cortex to motor neurons and interneurons; principal pathway for voluntary movement.

Spinothalamic tract. From the contralateral posterior horn to the thalamus; pain and temperature and some touch information from the contralateral half of the body.

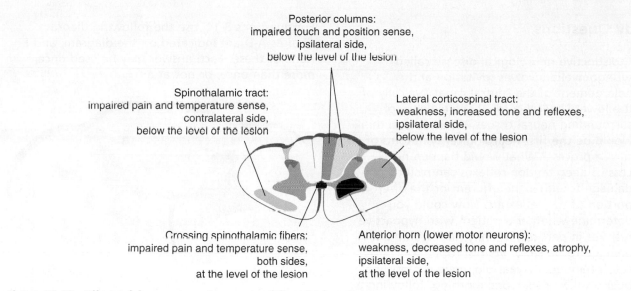

Posterior columns:
impaired touch and position sense,
ipsilateral side,
below the level of the lesion

Spinothalamic tract:
impaired pain and temperature sense,
contralateral side,
below the level of the lesion

Lateral corticospinal tract:
weakness, increased tone and reflexes,
ipsilateral side,
below the level of the lesion

Crossing spinothalamic fibers:
impaired pain and temperature sense,
both sides,
at the level of the lesion

Anterior horn (lower motor neurons):
weakness, decreased tone and reflexes, atrophy,
ipsilateral side,
at the level of the lesion

Figure 10-10   Effects of damage in various parts of the spinal cord.

partial cord damage (Fig. 10-10). Sensory deficits will be on the side ipsilateral to the damage if a pathway is affected before it crosses (e.g., posterior column), and on the contralateral side if affected after it crosses (e.g., spinothalamic tract). Weakness will be on the side ipsilateral to the damage because (1) lower motor neurons project to ipsilateral muscles, and (2) most corticospinal fibers cross in the pyramidal decussation (at the spinal cord-medulla junction) and are therefore on their way to ipsilateral lower motor neurons. So after unilateral damage there's a seemingly weird mix of ipsilateral (touch, position, strength) and contralateral (pain, temperature) deficits.

Study Questions

1. A distinctive neurological disease called syringomyelia involves cavitation and enlargement of the central canal, typically of the lower cervical cord, at the expense of surrounding neural tissues. What do you think would be the first neurological symptoms of such a process? What would happen next?

2. Loss of deep tendon reflexes can result from damage to either the afferent or the efferent portion of the reflex arc. How could you determine whether a patient with hypoactive reflexes in part of the body had suffered damage to dorsal or ventral roots?

3. A left-handed, 42-year-old, male professional beer drinker awoke one morning, following a strenuous workout with his team, with generalized weakness in the upper and lower extremities of both sides and pronounced bilateral deficits of pain and temperature sensibility on both sides of the body below the neck. There was no apparent disturbance of position sense, sensation of vibration, or tactile discrimination. Can you localize the problem anatomically?

For questions 4-7, choose the best match between the spinal levels in the column on the left and the contents in the column on the right.

4. C7	**a.**	does not exist.
5. C10	**b.**	contributes axons to the cauda equina.
6. T5	**c.**	contains preganglionic sympathetic neurons.
7. S3	**d.**	contains motor neurons for the upper extremity.

For questions 8-11, use the following diagram. Choices A-D are indicated on the diagram, and E = none of these. Each answer may be used once, more than once, or not at all.

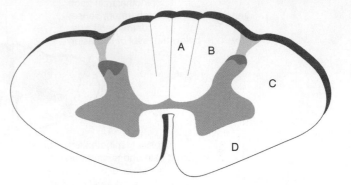

8. Arise from cell bodies in the contralateral posterior horn.
9. Branches of these fibers participate in the triceps stretch reflex.
10. These fibers have their cell bodies in contralateral dorsal root ganglia below T6.
11. Some of these fibers arise in the contralateral precentral gyrus.

12. The neural circuitry of the stretch reflex involves
    a. multiple interneurons in multiple spinal cord segments.
    b. small-diameter primary afferents.
    c. Golgi tendon organs.
    d. both a and c.
    e. none of the above.
13. Sympathetic motor neurons in the spinal cord
    a. have axons that end directly on smooth muscles.
    b. have axons that end in ganglia near or within smooth muscles and glands.
    c. are typically involved in "fight or flight" types of activities.
    d. none of the above.

Organization of the Brainstem

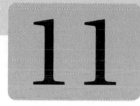

The Brainstem Has Conduit, Cranial Nerve, and Integrative Functions

The brainstem is another part of the CNS whose importance is out of proportion to its size. All the long tracts on their way to or from the spinal cord traverse the brainstem, so it has **conduit** functions. In addition, through connections with **cranial nerves** the brainstem takes care of the same basic sensory and motor functions for the head that the spinal cord does for the body, and takes care of some special senses as well (hearing, equilibrium, taste). Finally, the brainstem contains an anatomically diffuse **reticular formation** whose activity is crucial for a variety of functions, including the maintenance of consciousness.

The Medulla, Pons, and Midbrain Have Characteristic Gross Anatomical Features

Key Concepts

The medulla includes pyramids, olives, and part of the fourth ventricle.

The pons includes the basal pons, middle cerebellar peduncles, and part of the fourth ventricle.

The midbrain includes the superior and inferior colliculi, the cerebral peduncles, and the cerebral aqueduct.

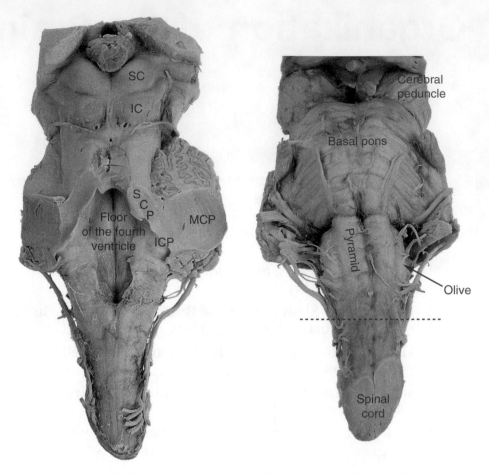

Figure 11-1   Major surface features of the brainstem. *IC*, Inferior colliculus; *ICP*, inferior cerebellar peduncle; *MCP*, middle cerebellar peduncle; *SC*, superior colliculus; *SCP*, superior cerebellar peduncle. The dashed line indicates the approximate transition from medulla to spinal cord. *(Thanks to Grant Dahmer.)*

Various nuclei and fiber bundles form surface features at different levels of the brainstem. The most prominent of these are listed in this section (Fig. 11-1).

Major surface features of the medulla include the **pyramids** and the **olives**. Each pyramid is a longitudinal bundle of fibers on the ventral surface of the medulla, made up of the corticospinal tract of that side of the brainstem. The olive is an ovoid bump dorsolateral to each pyramid in the rostral medulla, underlain by the **inferior olivary nucleus**, an important component of cerebellar circuitry. The central canal of the spinal cord continues into the medulla and opens up into the **fourth ventricle** at a mid-medullary level.

The pons is dominated by its basal part, a large transverse band of fibers and nuclei for which the pons is named (pons is Latin for "bridge"). The **basal pons** looks like it interconnects the two halves of the cerebellum, but instead it's the site of a transfer station through which each cerebral hemisphere talks to the contralateral half of the cerebellum. The **pontine nuclei** in each side of the basal pons receive cerebral inputs via the ipsilateral **corticopontine tract**. Axons from these nuclei then travel transversely, cross the midline, funnel into the contralateral **middle cerebellar peduncle**, and then fan out into the cerebellar cortex. The fourth ventricle is at its widest near the pontomedullary junction; it narrows progressively at more rostral pontine levels.

The surface of the midbrain includes the **inferior colliculi**, two rounded elevations on the dorsal surface of the caudal midbrain that are part of the auditory pathway; **superior colliculi**, two rounded elevations on the dorsal surface of the rostral midbrain, involved in eye movements and the direction of visual attention; and **cerebral peduncles**, large paired fiber bundles on the ventral surface of the midbrain, each carrying fibers descending from the cerebral cortex to the brainstem and spinal cord (mostly corticopontine and corticospinal fibers). The narrow fourth ventricle of the rostral pons is continuous with the cerebral aqueduct of the midbrain.

The Internal Structure of the Brainstem Reflects Surface Features and the Position of Long Tracts

Key Concepts

The corticospinal and spinothalamic tracts have consistent locations throughout the brainstem.

The medial lemniscus forms in the caudal medulla.

The rostral medulla contains the inferior olivary nucleus and part of the fourth ventricle.

The caudal pons is attached to the cerebellum by the middle cerebellar peduncle.

The superior cerebellar peduncle joins the brainstem in the rostral pons.

The superior cerebellar peduncles decussate in the caudal midbrain.

The rostral midbrain contains the red nucleus and substantia nigra.

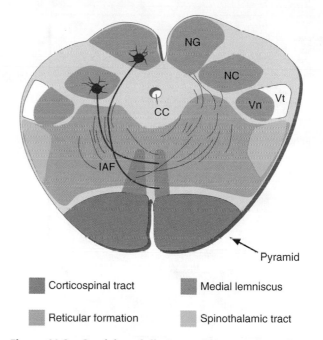

Figure 11-2   Caudal medulla (pyramids, central canal). As explained in Chapter 12, the spinal trigeminal tract and nucleus are the parts of the trigeminal system that take care of pain and temperature information from the head. *CC*, Central canal; *IAF*, internal arcuate fibers; *NC*, nucleus cuneatus; *NG*, nucleus gracilis; *Vn*, spinal trigeminal nucleus; *Vt*, spinal trigeminal tract.

The medulla, pons, and midbrain are commonly divided into rostral and caudal halves using some of the surface elevations just described and several other features. Each of these six brainstem levels has a few major, characteristic structures. All through the brainstem, the corticospinal tract is in a ventral location and the medial lemniscus is medial to the spinothalamic tract.

The **caudal** or **closed medulla** is the part that does not contain any portion of the fourth ventricle (Fig. 11-2); it extends from the pyramidal decussation to the beginning of the fourth ventricle. The posterior columns start to terminate in nuclei gracilis and cuneatus in the caudal medulla; axons of these second-order neurons arch through the reticular formation as **internal arcuate fibers**, cross the midline, and turn upstream as the medial lemniscus. The **rostral** or **open medulla** is the part that contains a portion of the fourth ventricle (Fig. 11-3); it extends from the caudal end of the fourth ventricle to the point at which the brainstem becomes attached to the cerebellum by the inferior and middle cerebellar peduncles. The pyramids are still there, and now the inferior olivary nucleus gets added. Axons of these neurons curve across the midline as more internal arcuate fibers and form most (but not nearly all) of the **inferior cerebellar peduncle**, which turns up into the cerebellum right at the pontomedullary junction.

Every level of the pons contains part of the basal pons and fourth ventricle; the **caudal pons** is the part physically attached to the cerebellum, primarily by the middle cerebellar peduncles (Fig. 11-4). Here the medial lemniscus starts to flatten out and move laterally, and axons

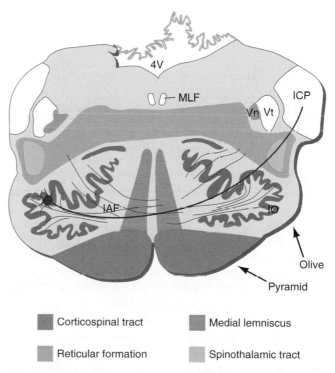

Figure 11-3   Rostral medulla (pyramids, fourth ventricle). *4V*, Fourth ventricle; *IAF*, internal arcuate fibers; *ICP*, inferior cerebellar peduncle; *IO*, inferior olivary nucleus; *MLF*, medial longitudinal fasciculus (explained in Chapter 12); *Vn*, spinal trigeminal nucleus; *Vt*, spinal trigeminal tract.

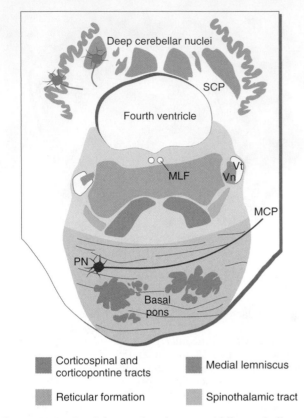

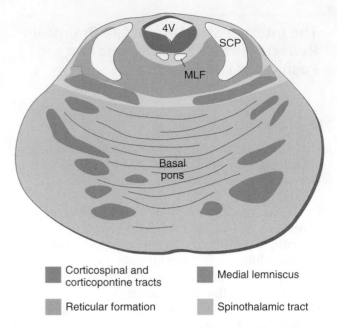

Figure 11-4 Caudal pons (basal pons, middle cerebellar peduncle). *MCP*, Middle cerebellar peduncle; *MLF*, medial longitudinal fasciculus; *PN*, pontine nuclei (clumps of gray matter scattered all through the basal pons, just one neuron shown here); *SCP*, superior cerebellar peduncle; *Vn*, spinal trigeminal nucleus; *Vt*, spinal trigeminal tract.

Figure 11-5 Rostral pons (basal pons, no attachment to cerebellum). *4V*, Fourth ventricle; *MLF*, medial longitudinal fasciculus; *SCP*, superior cerebellar peduncle.

emerging from **deep cerebellar nuclei** start to form the **superior cerebellar peduncle**. The **rostral pons** is no longer connected to the cerebellum (Fig. 11-5); the middle cerebellar peduncles haven't formed yet, and the superior cerebellar peduncles have left the cerebellum and are traveling rostrally through the brainstem. The trigeminal nerve is attached to the brainstem at the caudal pons-rostral pons junction.

The cerebral aqueduct continues the ventricular system through the midbrain, surrounded by a distinctive area of **periaqueductal gray** that participates in many of the autonomic control functions discussed in Chapter 23. The **caudal midbrain** is the part containing the inferior colliculi (Fig. 11-6). Here the superior cerebellar peduncles decussate, so inputs to the cerebellum from each cerebral hemisphere cross in the basal pons and outputs cross back in this **decussation of the superior cerebellar peduncles**. The **rostral midbrain** is the part containing the superior colliculi (Fig. 11-7); it also contains two other distinctive areas of gray matter, the **red nucleus** and **substantia nigra**. The red nucleus is hooked up in cerebellar circuitry (see Chapter 20), and the substantia nigra is part of the basal ganglia (see Chapter 19). The trochlear nerve emerges at the pons-

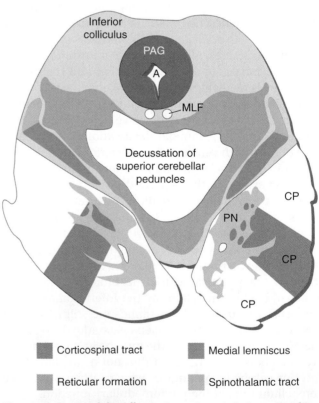

Figure 11-6 Caudal midbrain (aqueduct, inferior colliculi). *A*, Cerebral aqueduct; *CP*, cerebral peduncle (the middle part contains the corticospinal tract, most of the rest contains corticopontine fibers); *MLF*, medial longitudinal fasciculus; *PAG*, periaqueductal gray; *PN*, pontine nuclei (the last few, as the cerebral peduncles replace the basal pons).

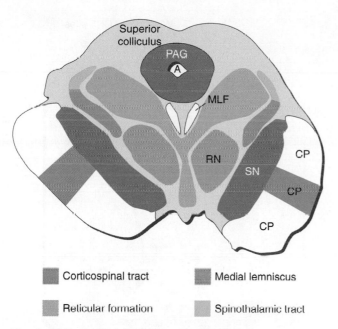

Superior colliculus

PAG

A

MLF

RN

SN

CP

CP

CP

■ Corticospinal tract   ■ Medial lemniscus

■ Reticular formation   ■ Spinothalamic tract

Figure 11-7 Rostral midbrain (aqueduct, superior colliculi). *A*, Cerebral aqueduct; *CP*, cerebral peduncle; *MLF*, medial longitudinal fasciculus; *PAG*, periaqueductal gray; *RN*, red nucleus (the superior cerebellar peduncles seem to have disappeared, but their fibers mostly pass through or around this nucleus); *SN*, substantia nigra.

midbrain junction, and the posterior commissure is located at the midbrain-diencephalon junction.

Figures 11-2 through 11-7 indicate just the major features of each of these brainstem levels. Information about additional brainstem functions and connections (e.g., cranial nerve nuclei) can be found in THB6 and in Chapters 12-14 of this book. The same figures are shown again in Chapter 15, with the structures discussed in Chapters 12-14 added in.

The Reticular Core of the Brainstem Is Involved in Multiple Functions

Key Concepts

The reticular formation participates in the control of movement through connections with both the spinal cord and the cerebellum.
The reticular formation modulates the transmission of information in pain pathways.
The reticular formation contains autonomic reflex circuitry.
The reticular formation is involved in the control of arousal and consciousness.

The reticular formation forms a core of neural tissue in the brainstem, surrounded by cranial nerve nuclei and the tracts mentioned thus far. It samples the information carried by most sensory, motor, and visceral pathways. The reticular formation uses some of this information in various reflexes (e.g., circulatory and respiratory reflexes, swallowing, coughing). It also sends outputs caudally to the spinal cord and rostrally to the diencephalon and cerebral cortex. The outputs to the spinal cord mediate some aspects of movement, control the sensitivity of spinal reflexes, and regulate the transmission of sensory information (especially pain) into ascending pathways. The outputs to the cerebrum from a portion of the reticular formation called the **ascending reticular activating system** (**ARAS**) modulate the level of cortical activity and hence the level of consciousness; the ARAS is important in sleep-wake cycles.

Some Brainstem Nuclei Have Distinctive Neurochemical Signatures

Most of the neurons described so far in this book have discrete connections that seem to suit them for preserving the details of information—e.g., somatotopic projections from motor cortex to lower motor neurons, or from nucleus cuneatus to a particular small part of the thalamus. In contrast, there are some collections of brainstem neurons with extremely widespread connections, not designed for point-to-point transmission of information, but designed instead to have **modulatory** effects that regulate the background level of activity in large parts of the CNS. Each of these collections is made up of neurons using a distinctive small-molecule transmitter with slow, second-messenger effects on their targets. The most prominent examples are norepinephrine, dopamine, serotonin, and acetylcholine. The diffuse projections of the central **noradrenergic**, **dopaminergic**, **serotonergic**, and **cholinergic** neurons make them better suited for more general roles in adjusting the background level of activity or sensitivity of large parts of the CNS, each of the four in a somewhat different way.

Neurons of the Locus Ceruleus Contain Norepinephrine

Neurons that use norepinephrine as a transmitter (noradrenergic neurons) are found in the peripheral nervous system as postganglionic sympathetic neurons. In the CNS, some are located in the medullary reticular formation, but most are pigmented neurons of the **locus ceruleus** in the rostral pons (Fig. 11-8). CNS noradrenergic neurons collectively project to practically every part of the CNS.

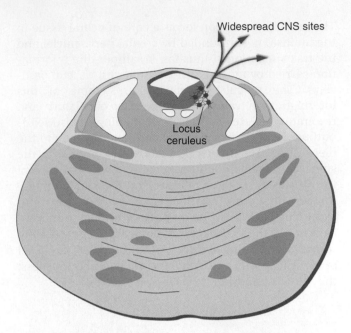

Figure 11-8 Noradrenergic neurons of the locus ceruleus.

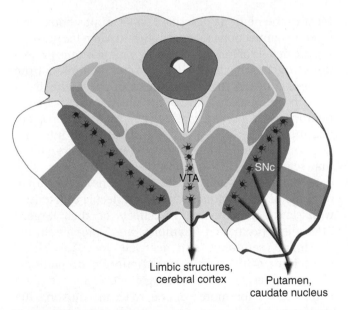

Figure 11-9 Brainstem dopaminergic neurons. As discussed in Chapter 19, the substantia nigra is a two-part structure. The part farther from the cerebral peduncle (the compact part) is where the dopaminergic neurons live. *SNc*, Substantia nigra (compact part); *VTA*, ventral tegmental area.

Neurons of the Substantia Nigra and Ventral Tegmental Area Contain Dopamine

Most of the neurons that use dopamine as a transmitter (dopaminergic neurons) are located in the midbrain (Fig. 11-9), either in the **compact part** of the **substantia nigra** or closer to the midline in the **ventral tegmental area**. Nigral dopaminergic neurons project to the caudate nucleus and putamen, and their degeneration causes

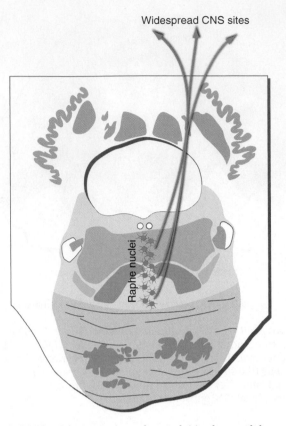

Figure 11-10 Serotonergic raphe nuclei in the caudal pons. Similar serotonergic neurons are distributed in midline raphe nuclei in most of the brainstem.

Parkinson's disease. Ventral tegmental neurons project to an assortment of limbic structures and (mostly frontal) cortical areas, and malfunction of these neurons or their targets plays a role in some forms of mental illness.

Neurons of the Raphe Nuclei Contain Serotonin

Neurons that use serotonin as a transmitter (serotonergic neurons) are located primarily in the **raphe nuclei**, a collective name for a series of nuclei near the midline of the brainstem reticular formation (Fig. 11-10). Like the noradrenergic neurons of the locus ceruleus, the serotonergic neurons of the raphe nuclei project practically everywhere in the CNS, suggesting that they too may be involved in adjusting levels of attention or arousal.

Neurons of the Rostral Brainstem and Basal Forebrain Contain Acetylcholine

Neurons that use acetylcholine as a transmitter (cholinergic neurons) play an important role in the peripheral nervous system. Some are located entirely in the periphery (postganglionic parasympathetic neurons), whereas others have their cell bodies in the CNS and axons that

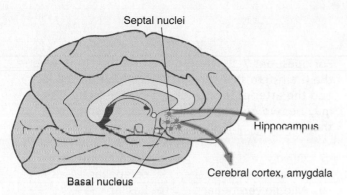

Figure 11-11 CNS cholinergic neurons in the basal nucleus. Other cholinergic neurons in the midbrain reticular formation modulate the activity of the thalamus.

travel through spinal or cranial nerves (lower motor neurons, preganglionic sympathetic and parasympathetic neurons).

Some CNS cholinergic neurons are local interneurons in various structures (such as the putamen and caudate nucleus). Others have longer axons that project from one part of the CNS to another. Some of these are located in the midbrain reticular formation, but the largest collection is in the **basal nucleus (of Meynert)**, a group of large cholinergic neurons in the basal forebrain (Fig. 11-11) that project to widespread areas of the cerebral cortex. Nearby cholinergic neurons in the **septal nuclei** project to the hippocampus. These basal forebrain neurons degenerate in victims of Alzheimer's disease.

The Brainstem Is Supplied by the Vertebral-Basilar System

The vertebral arteries run along the lateral and anterior surfaces of the medulla and fuse to form the basilar artery, which runs along the anterior surface of the pons until it bifurcates into the posterior cerebral arteries on the anterior surface of the midbrain (THB6 Figures 6-3

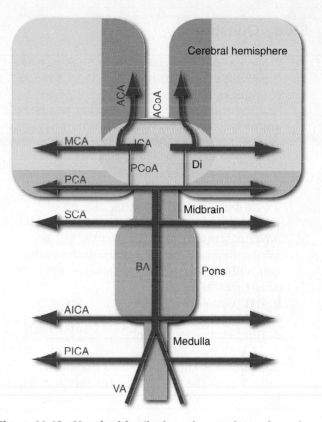

Figure 11-12 Vertebral-basilar branches on the surface of the brainstem. *ACA*, Anterior cerebral artery; *ACoA*, anterior communicating artery; *AICA*, anterior inferior cerebellar artery; *BA*, basilar artery; *Di*, diencephalon; *ICA*, internal carotid artery; *PCA*, posterior cerebral artery; *PCoA*, posterior communicating artery; *PICA*, posterior inferior cerebellar artery; *SCA*, superior cerebellar artery; *VA*, vertebral artery.

and 11-29, pp. 126 and 291). Hence, nearly the entire supply of the brainstem comes from the vertebral-basilar posterior cerebral system (THB6 Figure 11-30, p. 292). Knowing where each of the major branches from this system arises lets you surmise the supply of different levels of the brainstem (Fig. 11-12), because even if a branch (e.g., PICA) is headed for someplace like the cerebellum it needs to wrap around the brainstem to get there.

Study Questions

1. A 39-year-old hypertensive handball hustler, in the midst of a shouting match with a much younger opponent (who was losing badly), had the sudden onset of a searing headache and briefly lost consciousness. When he awoke, his left arm and leg were numb and somewhat weak, he had a Babinski sign on the left, and movements of his left arm and leg were grossly uncoordinated (more than would be expected from the degree of weakness). He was later determined by MRI to have suffered a brainstem stroke, but an astute medical student watching the match had already surmised that damage was in the
   a. left rostral medulla.
   b. left rostral midbrain.
   c. right rostral medulla.
   d. right rostral midbrain.

For questions 2-6, choose the best match between the structures in the column on the left and the brainstem levels in the column on the right.

2. Red nucleus
3. Inferior colliculus
4. Nucleus gracilis
5. Inferior olivary nucleus
6. Decussation of superior cerebellar peduncles

   a. Caudal medulla
   b. Rostral medulla
   c. Caudal pons
   d. Caudal midbrain
   e. Rostral midbrain

For questions 7-11, choose the best match between the brainstem structures in the column on the left and the arteries in the column on the right. (There may be two equally good matches for some of these.)

7. Olive
8. Basal pons
9. Middle cerebellar peduncle
10. Cerebral peduncle
11. Inferior cerebellar peduncle

   a. Anterior inferior cerebellar
   b. Basilar
   c. Posterior cerebral
   d. Posterior inferior cerebellar
   e. Superior cerebellar
   f. Vertebral

Answer questions 12-15 using the following list. Each item may be used once, more than once, or not at all.

   a. Acetylcholine
   b. Dopamine
   c. Norepinephrine
   d. Serotonin
   e. Glutamate
   f. GABA

12. Implicated in Parkinson's disease.
13. Synthesized mainly by neurons with their cell bodies near the midline throughout the brainstem reticular formation.
14. Used as a transmitter by neurons of the locus ceruleus.
15. Used as a transmitter by neurons that project from the basal nucleus to widespread cortical areas.

Cranial Nerves and Their Nuclei

12

Cranial nerves and their central connections often look bewilderingly complicated, but for the most part they are actually arranged systematically.

Cranial Nerve Nuclei Have a Generally Predictable Arrangement

Key Concept

The sulcus limitans intervenes between motor and sensory nuclei of cranial nerves.

The olfactory nerve (I) is a series of thin filaments that attach directly to the olfactory bulb, part of the telencephalon. Fibers of the optic nerve (II) proceed through the optic chiasm and tract (see Chapter 17), and most end in the lateral geniculate nucleus of the thalamus, part of the diencephalon. The 10 remaining cranial nerves originate or terminate in the brainstem (or upper cervical spinal cord), as indicated in Table 12-1 and Fig. 12-1. The taste afferents in the **facial**, **glossopharyngeal**, and **vagus nerves** (**VII, IX, X**) are considered separately in Chapter 13, along with the olfactory nerve (I), and the **vestibulocochlear nerve** (**VIII**) has its own chapter (14). The

Table 12-1	Major functions of the brainstem cranial nerves	
Cranial Nerve	**Main Functions**	**Attachment Point**
III. Oculomotor	Eye movements, pupil, lens	Rostral midbrain (V)
IV. Trochlear	Eye movements (superior oblique)	Pons/midbrain junction (D)
V. Trigeminal	Facial sensation, chewing	Midpons (L)
VI. Abducens	Eye movements (lateral rectus)	Pontomedullary junction (V)
VII. Facial	Facial expression, taste	Pontomedullary junction (V/L)
VIII. Vestibulocochlear	Hearing, equilibrium	Pontomedullary junction (V/L)
IX. Glossopharyngeal	Taste, swallowing	Rostral medulla (L)
X. Vagus	Visceral sensory Speaking, swallowing Preganglionic parasympathetic	Rostral medulla (L)
XI. Accessory	Head and shoulder movement	Upper cervical spinal cord (L)
XII. Hypoglossal	Tongue movement	Rostral medulla (V/L)

D, *L*, and *V* indicate dorsal, lateral, and ventral attachment points.

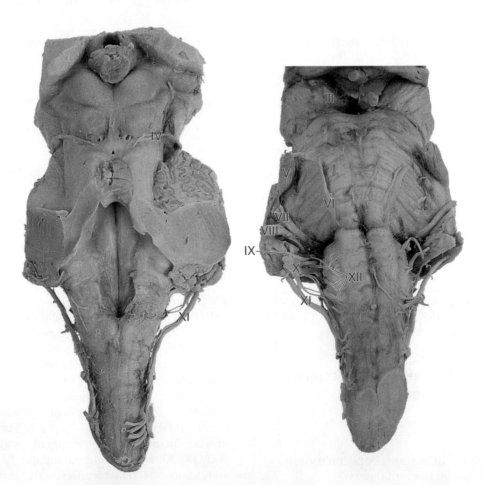

Figure 12-1   Attachment points of cranial nerves III-XII. *(Thanks to Grant Dahmer.)*

rest of the brainstem cranial nerves are introduced in this chapter.

The wiring principles discussed in Chapter 3 and applied to the spinal cord in Chapter 10 also apply, for the most part, to cranial nerves and their connections. At its attachment point, each brainstem cranial nerve is carrying sensory information from ipsilateral receptors or motor output to ipsilateral muscles (except for the case of afferents and efferents for places like abdominal viscera, where the ipsilateral-contralateral concept loses much of its meaning). Thus, the right vestibulocochlear nerve (VIII) carries information from the right cochlea and the left **oculomotor nerve (III)** innervates muscles of the left eye. Similarly, the fibers of these cranial nerves mostly terminate in or originate from the ipsilateral side of the CNS. The principal exceptions are the **trochlear (IV)** and oculomotor nerves. All trochlear fibers and some oculomotor fibers originate from motor neurons in the contralateral half of the CNS.

Some fairly simple rules can be used to predict the approximate locations of cranial nerve nuclei—collections of second-order sensory neurons, lower motor neurons, and preganglionic parasympathetic neurons. The medial-lateral location of a nucleus is predicted by the **sulcus limitans**, and the longitudinal location by the level of attachment of the cranial nerve associated with it (Fig. 12-2). Sensory nuclei are typically located lateral to the sulcus limitans and motor nuclei medial to it because of the way the neural tube opens up at the level

of the fourth ventricle. Visceral nuclei are located closer to the sulcus limitans, so for example second-order taste neurons are just lateral to the sulcus limitans and visceral motor (= preganglionic parasympathetic) neurons just medial to it.

Cranial Nerves III, IV, VI, and XII Contain Somatic Motor Fibers

Key Concepts

The oculomotor nerve (III) innervates four of the six extraocular muscles.

The trochlear nerve (IV) innervates the superior oblique.

The abducens nerve (VI) innervates the lateral rectus.

The oculomotor (III), trochlear (IV), **abducens (VI)**, and **hypoglossal (XII)** nerves are the simplest cranial nerves, in the sense that they just contain motor axons to ordinary skeletal muscle (except for some clinically important parasympathetics in the oculomotor nerve).

The trochlear nerve (IV) innervates the superior oblique muscle and the abducens nerve (VI) innervates

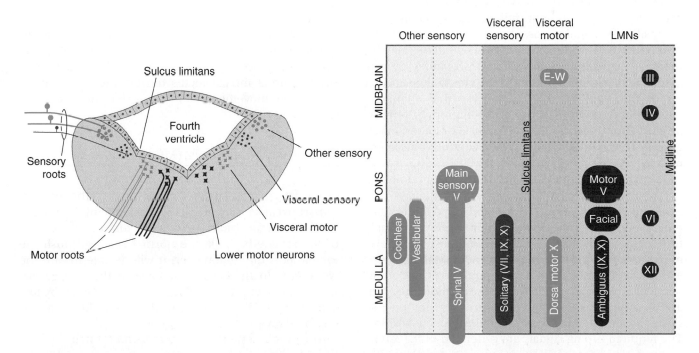

Figure 12-2 Locations of cranial nerve nuclei. The general medial-lateral arrangement is shown on the left. The 2D grid on the right is a schematic view looking down on the left half of the brainstem; it shows the longitudinal and medial-lateral arrangement of the major cranial nerve nuclei discussed in this chapter (the accessory nucleus, in the upper cervical spinal cord, is omitted). *E-W*, Edinger-Westphal nucleus (part of the oculomotor nucleus).

the lateral rectus. The oculomotor nerve (III) innervates the remaining extraocular muscles (medial, superior, and inferior recti, inferior oblique) and the elevator of the eyelid, and it also contains the preganglionic parasympathetic fibers for the pupillary sphincter and the ciliary muscle. All three of these nerves, once they leave the brainstem, proceed to the ipsilateral eye (although trochlear and some oculomotor fibers cross before leaving the brainstem). The hypoglossal nerve (XII) innervates the muscles of the ipsilateral half of the tongue.

As expected from their embryological development, the oculomotor, trochlear, abducens, and hypoglossal nuclei are located near the midline in the floor of the ventricular system. The oculomotor nucleus is in the rostral midbrain (THB6 Figure 12-4, p. 301), the trochlear nucleus in the caudal midbrain (THB6 Figure 12-5, p. 302), the abducens nucleus in the caudal pons (THB6 Figure 12-6, p. 303), and the hypoglossal nucleus in the rostral medulla (THB6 Figure 12-11, p. 306).

The Abducens Nucleus Also Contains Interneurons That Project to the Contralateral Oculomotor Nucleus

Any time we look to the left or the right, we need to contract the lateral rectus of one eye and the medial rectus of the other eye simultaneously. Theoretically, this could be accomplished by having separate, parallel inputs to both sets of motor neurons. However, we have evolved a different mechanism to achieve the same end. The abducens nucleus contains not only the motor neurons for the ipsilateral lateral rectus, but also an equal number of interneurons whose axons cross the midline, join the **medial longitudinal fasciculus** (**MLF**), and ascend to medial rectus motor neurons in the contralateral oculomotor nucleus (Fig. 12-3). Anything that stimulates lateral rectus motor neurons during attempted horizontal gaze also stimulates the interneurons, so coordinated gaze is achieved when we try to contract one lateral rectus.

Inputs to the abducens nucleus arise in a number of sites, including the **vestibular nuclei.** (This allows us to generate eye movements equal and opposite to head movements—the **vestibulo-ocular reflex,** covered further in Chapter 14.) Ordinary voluntary eye movements are of a rapid type called **saccades**. Making a rapid eye movement over to a target requires a rapid initial burst of action potentials in abducens motor neurons and interneurons to get the eyes moving, followed by slower maintained firing to maintain the new position. The required timing signals are generated in the reticular formation near the abducens nucleus, a region called the **paramedian pontine reticular formation** (or **PPRF**, or **pontine gaze center**). Hence, damage to one abducens nucleus causes loss of all horizontal eye movements

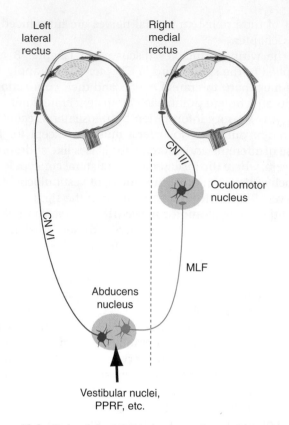

Figure 12-3 Role of the MLF in horizontal gaze. The MLF gets involved in the coordination of head and eye movements in other ways as well, but its content of abducens interneuron axons is the basis of its most prominent role.

to the ipsilateral side, but damage to the PPRF causes selective loss of rapid eye movements to the ipsilateral side. Damage to one MLF causes selective weakness of the ipsilateral medial rectus during attempted lateral gaze. (Eye movements are discussed more fully in Chapter 21.)

The Hypoglossal Nerve (XII) Innervates Tongue Muscles

A normal tongue when protruded stays in the midline, in part because the muscles of each side of the tongue push toward the midline with equal force. So if one side of the tongue is weak, the normal side will push the tongue past the midline and it will deviate toward the weak side. In the case of damage to the hypoglossal nerve or nucleus, the weakness is accompanied by fasciculations and atrophy, typical signs of lower motor neuron damage.

Upper motor neurons for tongue motor neurons, like those for spinal cord motor neurons, are located in the precentral gyrus and adjacent cortical areas. Their axons, called **corticobulbar** fibers, accompany corticospinal axons through the internal capsule, cerebral peduncle, and pons. In the rostral medulla, they leave the cortico-spinal fibers and end in the hypoglossal nucleus. As they do so, many but not all of them cross the midline. Hence, both sides of the tongue can be made to contract by one cerebral hemisphere, and unilateral damage to corti-cobulbar fibers does not cause profound or lasting weakness of either side of the tongue. However, most of us have substantially more crossed than uncrossed fibers, so there is often some transient weakness on the contra-lateral side following corticobulbar damage. In such a case, cortical damage would cause tongue deviation *away* from the side of the lesion because the weak side would be contralateral to the lesion.

Branchiomeric Nerves Contain Axons from Multiple Categories

The **trigeminal (V)**, **facial (VII)**, **glossopharyngeal (IX)**, **vagus (X)**, and **accessory (XI)** nerves are more complex than the ones considered so far. Each innervates skeletal muscle derived embryologically from the **branchial arches**. Except for the accessory nerve, each innervates other things, too. Nevertheless, each has only one or two major functions (see Table 12-1 at the beginning of this chapter).

The Trigeminal Nerve (V) Is the General Sensory Nerve for the Head

The trigeminal nerve (V) is the principal somatosensory nerve for the head, with afferents arriving through its ophthalmic, maxillary, and mandibular divisions (THB6 Figure 12-13, p. 307). The afferent fibers have cell bodies in the **trigeminal ganglion** (except for a few, mainly from muscle spindles, whose cell bodies are inside the CNS in the **mesencephalic nucleus of the trigeminal nerve**, located in the rostral pons and extending into the mid-brain). Central processes of all trigeminal primary afferents end either in the **main sensory nucleus**, located in the midpons, or in the **spinal trigeminal nucleus**, which merges rostrally with the main sensory nucleus and cau-dally with the posterior horn of the upper cervical spinal cord. Fibers headed for the spinal trigeminal nucleus get there by traveling just lateral to it, through the **spinal trigeminal tract**.

Motor neurons for the masseter and several smaller muscles are located in the **trigeminal motor nucleus**, medial to the main sensory nucleus in the midpons.

The Main Sensory Nucleus Receives Information about Touch and Jaw Position

Large-diameter trigeminal afferents, carrying informa-tion about touch and jaw position, end in the main

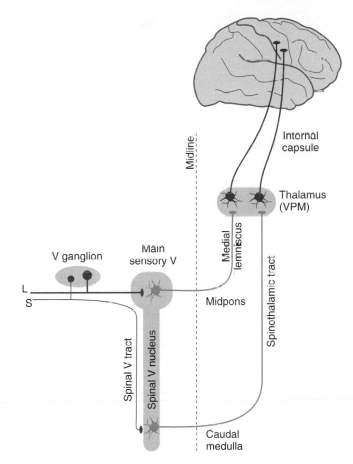

Figure 12-4 Trigeminal sensory connections. (Although all trigeminal primary afferents are indicated as having cell bodies in the trigeminal ganglion, some of those with large-diameter axons actually live in the mesencephalic nucleus.) *L*, Large-diameter fibers; *S*, small-diameter fibers.

sensory nucleus (Fig. 12-4). The main sensory nucleus is the trigeminal equivalent of a posterior column nucleus. Second-order fibers from the main sensory nucleus cross the midline, join the medial lemniscus, and reach the ventral posteromedial nucleus (VPM) of the thala-mus. VPM neurons then project to somatosensory cortex of the postcentral gyrus and adjacent areas. In contrast to the situation in the spinal cord, large-diameter tri-geminal afferents do not travel through anything com-parable to the posterior columns before reaching their nucleus of termination (Fig. 12-5).

The Spinal Trigeminal Nucleus Receives Information about Pain and Temperature

Small-diameter trigeminal afferents, carrying pain and temperature and some touch information, turn caudally in the spinal trigeminal tract. The pain and temperature fibers end in portions of the spinal trigeminal nucleus in the caudal medulla and upper cervical spinal cord.

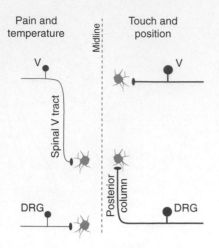

Figure 12-5 Locations of second-order neurons in trigeminal and spinal sensory pathways. *DRG*, Dorsal root ganglion; *V*, trigeminal ganglion.

Second-order fibers from the spinal trigeminal nucleus then cross the midline, join the spinothalamic tract, and reach VPM and other thalamic nuclei (see Fig. 12-4). Thalamic neurons then project to somatosensory cortex of the postcentral gyrus and other areas. In contrast to the situation in the spinal cord, small-diameter trigeminal afferents travel an appreciable distance through the CNS (in the spinal trigeminal tract) before reaching the second-order neurons on which they terminate (see Fig. 12-5).

The primary afferent fibers in the spinal trigeminal tract are arranged somatotopically (Fig. 12-6), with the ipsilateral half of the face represented upside down

(i.e., ophthalmic division fibers most ventral, mandibular division fibers most dorsal). In addition to this dorsal-ventral gradient, there is a rostral-caudal order in which the pain and temperature fibers terminate in the spinal trigeminal nucleus. Fibers representing areas near the midline terminate most rostrally (i.e., in the mid-medulla), and fibers representing more lateral areas terminate most caudally (i.e., in the upper cervical spinal cord). This makes sense because it means that pain and temperature afferents from the back of the head (i.e., upper cervical dorsal roots) end near the termination sites of trigeminal afferents from nearby areas of the head.

The rest of the spinal trigeminal nucleus (i.e., the parts in the rostral medulla and caudal pons) takes care of the remaining spinal-cord-like somatosensory functions for the head. These include things like getting trigeminal information to the cerebellum, as well as providing the interneurons for the blink reflex (see Fig. 12-8), which is a trigeminal equivalent of a withdrawal reflex.

The Trigeminal Motor Nucleus Innervates Muscles of Mastication

Trigeminal motor neurons are involved not just in routine chewing, but also in a **jaw-jerk reflex** (Fig. 12-7) homologous to the knee-jerk reflex: stretching the masseter causes a reflex contraction by way of a monosynaptic circuit parallel to that of spinal stretch reflexes. The afferent cell bodies for this reflex are peculiar in that they reside within the CNS (in the mesencephalic trigeminal nucleus).

Figure 12-6 Somatotopy in the spinal trigeminal system, as it would be seen in cross sections of the spinal trigeminal tract and nucleus (SpV) in the mid-medulla and caudal medulla.

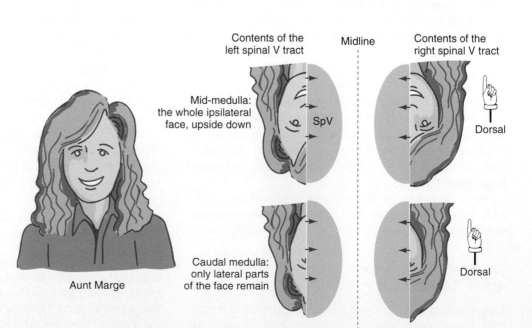

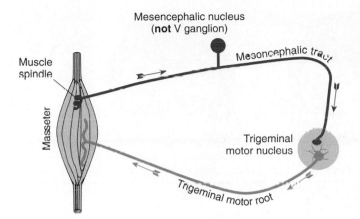

Figure 12-7 The jaw-jerk reflex arc. Just as in the case of spinal primary afferents, these trigeminal primary afferents have additional branches that end in trigeminal sensory nuclei.

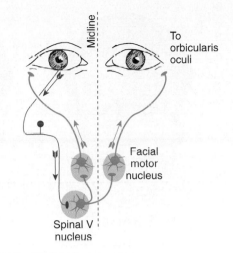

Figure 12-8 Blink reflex circuitry.

Key Concept

The facial (VII), glossopharyngeal (IX), and vagus (X) nerves all contain somatic and visceral sensory, visceral motor, and branchial motor fibers.

The Facial Nerve (VII) Innervates Muscles of Facial Expression

A major component of the facial nerve (VII) is the axons of the motor neurons for the muscles of facial expression (and the stapedius, a small but important middle ear muscle). These originate in the **facial motor nucleus** of the caudal pons, but loop around the abducens nucleus as the **internal genu** of the facial nerve before leaving the brainstem to innervate the ipsilateral half of the face (THB6 Figure 12-7, p. 303).

The jaw-jerk reflex is the only prominent monosynaptic cranial nerve reflex. Other brainstem reflexes, like other spinal reflexes, involve interneurons. Many of these reflexes are protective in nature, like the spinal flexor (withdrawal) reflex. An example is blinking both eyes when an object touches either cornea. The afferents for this **blink reflex** (Fig. 12-8) travel in the trigeminal nerve, the efferents (cell bodies in the facial motor nucleus) in the facial nerve.

Upper Motor Neuron Damage Affects the Upper and Lower Parts of the Face Differently

Corticobulbar fibers to the motor neurons for the lower half of the face are mostly crossed, corresponding to the way we can move both sides of the lower face relatively independently. However, corticobulbar fibers to the motor neurons for the upper half of the face are distrib-

uted bilaterally, corresponding to the way both sides of the upper face usually move together. Hence, all parts of the face except the ipsilateral lower quadrant can be made to contract by one cerebral hemisphere, and so unilateral corticobulbar damage causes weakness of only the contralateral lower quadrant (Fig. 12-9). (For example, after left motor cortex damage the intact right hemisphere cannot make the muscles of the right lower quadrant contract.) In contrast, unilateral damage to the facial nerve or nucleus causes weakness of the entire ipsilateral half of the face.

The Vagus Nerve (X) Is the Principal Parasympathetic Nerve

Key Concept

The glossopharyngeal nerve (IX) conveys information from intraoral receptors.

Afferent fibers from the thoracic and abdominal viscera reach the brainstem with the vagus nerve. They travel within the brainstem in the **solitary tract** of the rostral medulla and end in the surrounding **nucleus of the solitary tract** (Fig. 12-10). A smaller number of glossopharyngeal afferents, mostly from the mouth and throat, follow a similar course in the CNS. Neurons in the nucleus of the solitary tract participate in various visceral reflexes (e.g., automatic adjustment of respiratory and cardiovascular functions) and also convey information directly or indirectly to the hypothalamus and thalamus.

Motor neurons for the muscles of the larynx and pharynx are located in the reticular formation of the rostral medulla, just dorsal to the inferior olivary nucleus, as **nucleus ambiguus**. Most of them travel peripherally

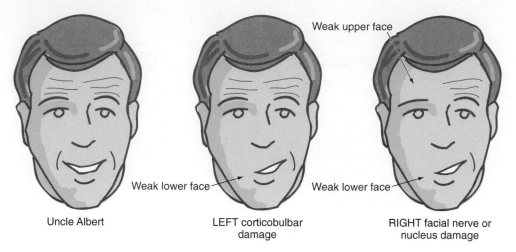

Weak upper face

Weak lower face

Weak lower face

Uncle Albert

LEFT corticobulbar damage

RIGHT facial nerve or nucleus damage

Figure 12-9 Patterns of facial weakness following upper motor neuron or lower motor neuron damage (supranuclear vs. nuclear facial palsy, respectively).

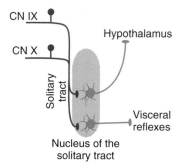

CN IX

CN X

Hypothalamus

Solitary tract

Visceral reflexes

Nucleus of the solitary tract

Figure 12-10 Visceral connections of the nucleus of the solitary tract. (As discussed in Chapter 13, this nucleus also has a critical role in taste.)

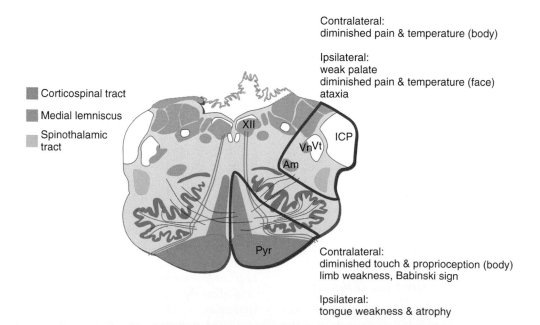

Contralateral:
diminished pain & temperature (body)

Ipsilateral:
weak palate
diminished pain & temperature (face)
ataxia

Corticospinal tract

Medial lemniscus

Spinothalamic tract

XII

ICP

VnVt

Am

Pyr

Contralateral:
diminished touch & proprioception (body)
limb weakness, Babinski sign

Ipsilateral:
tongue weakness & atrophy

Figure 12-11 Lesions and symptoms of the medial and lateral medullary syndromes, two examples of crossed syndromes. These could be caused by occlusion of a branch of the vertebral or posterior inferior cerebellar arteries, respectively. *Am*, Nucleus ambiguus; *ICP*, inferior cerebellar peduncle; *Pyr*, pyramid; *Vn* and *Vt*, spinal trigeminal nucleus and tract; *XII*, hypoglossal nucleus.

in the vagus nerve (X) to ipsilateral muscles; a few travel in the glossopharyngeal nerve (IX).

Corticobulbar fibers to nucleus ambiguus are distributed bilaterally, so unilateral corticobulbar damage usually causes no serious long-term laryngeal or pharyngeal deficits.

The principal collection of preganglionic parasympathetic neurons in the brainstem is the **dorsal motor nucleus** of the vagus nerve, located just lateral to the hypoglossal nucleus in the rostral medulla. Their axons travel through the vagus nerve to ganglia that innervate the thoracic and abdominal viscera. A few others travel from more rostral brainstem sites with the glossopharyngeal nerve (→parotid gland), the facial nerve (→salivary and lacrimal glands), and the oculomotor nerve (→pupillary sphincter and ciliary muscle).

The Accessory Nerve (XI) Innervates Neck and Shoulder Muscles

The **accessory nucleus**, in the upper cervical spinal cord, contains the lower motor neurons for the trapezius and sternocleidomastoid, so damage here or in the accessory nerve (XI) causes problems shrugging the ipsilateral shoulder or turning the head to the contralateral side.

Brainstem Damage Commonly Causes Deficits on One Side of the Head and the Opposite Side of the Body

Once the medial lemniscus has formed, all the major long tracts in the brainstem are related to the contralateral side of the body. In contrast, fibers entering or leaving the brainstem in cranial nerves are hooked up to ipsilateral structures. The result is that damage on one side of the brainstem causes contralateral problems in the body, but ipsilateral problems in the head (Fig. 12-11). These kinds of **crossed findings** are hard to produce with damage anyplace else in the nervous system and are usually a dead giveaway that it's a brainstem lesion. Knowing the locations of the long tracts and of cranial nerve attachment levels often lets you localize brainstem damage with amazing precision.

Study Questions

For questions 1-4, choose the most likely site of damage from the following list.

LEFT	RIGHT
a. Medulla	**d.** Medulla
b. Pons	**e.** Pons
c. Midbrain	**f.** Midbrain

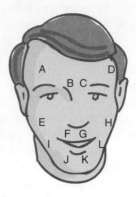

1. A beleaguered 39-year-old handball player with a drooping right eyelid, laterally deviated right eye, dilated right pupil, weak left arm and leg, and left Babinski sign.
2. A patient with a weak right arm and leg, right Babinski sign, and impaired touch and position sense in the right arm and leg. Her tongue deviates to the left when protruded.
3. A patient with a weak left arm and leg, left Babinski sign, and impaired touch and position sense in the left arm and leg. His right eye is deviated medially, and his tongue deviates slightly to the left when protruded.
4. A patient with diminished pain and temperature sensation over the right arm and leg and the left side of the face, ataxic left arm and leg, and a palate whose left side does not elevate when he says "Ahhhhh."

5. The trigeminal nerve contains all of the following *except*
    a. motor axons to the masseter.
    b. primary afferents carrying gustatory information from taste buds in the back of the tongue.
    c. primary afferents carrying pain and temperature information from the forehead.
    d. primary afferents that end in the main sensory nucleus in the midpons.
    e. primary afferents from masseter muscle spindles.
6. Primary afferent fibers conveying pain and temperature information from the left side of the forehead terminate
    a. bilaterally in the spinal trigeminal nucleus.
    b. in the main sensory nucleus of the trigeminal nerve on the left side.
    c. in the spinal trigeminal nucleus of the left side.
    d. in VPM of the thalamus on the right side.
7. Do the relative positions of the trigeminal motor and main sensory nuclei make embryological sense?
8. The most ventral fibers of the left spinal trigeminal tract at the spinomedullary junction represent which of the following areas?

9. Interruption of corticobulbar fibers in the left cerebral peduncle would result in weakness of
    a. the left side of the face.
    b. the right side of the face.
    c. the left lower quadrant of the face.
    d. the right lower quadrant of the face.
    e. the upper half of the face.
10. Motor neurons for the skeletal muscles of the larynx and pharynx are located in (the)
    a. dorsal motor nucleus of the vagus.
    b. nucleus ambiguus.
    c. nucleus of the solitary tract.
    d. trigeminal motor nucleus.
    e. facial motor nucleus.
11. Preganglionic parasympathetic fibers leave the brainstem in all of the following cranial nerves *except*
    a. III.
    b. V.
    c. VII.
    d. IX.
    e. X.
12. The nerve fibers of the solitary tract
    a. are central branches of facial, glossopharyngeal, and hypoglossal fibers.
    b. convey gustatory and olfactory chemosensory information.
    c. mostly terminate in nucleus ambiguus.
    d. serve as the afferent limb of a variety of reflexes, including those that modulate cardiac and respiratory function.
13. Given that a patient had suffered damage to *either* one trigeminal nerve or one facial nerve, how could you determine which nerve was affected (and on which side), using one stroke of a wisp of cotton?
14. Trigeminal neuralgia is a condition of severe, intermittent pain in part of the trigeminal distribution. Total destruction of the trigeminal ganglion has been used as a treatment for this condition. What practical complications might arise from this treatment?

The Chemical Senses of Taste and Smell

13

The Perception of Flavor Involves Gustatory, Olfactory, Trigeminal, and Other Inputs

When we eat food or drink a beverage, we have a unified perception, centered on the tongue, of some mixture of flavors. However, this unified perception actually results from the CNS combining multiple kinds of information—somatosensory inputs reflecting things like temperature, texture, and fizziness, as well as inputs about the chemical makeup of the food

from three different sources. Chemicals dissolved in the mouth stimulate taste buds, providing **gustatory** information. Simultaneously, vapors emanating from the food reach **olfactory receptor cells** through either the nostrils or the oropharynx (THB6 Figure 13-8, p. 330). Finally, some dissolved chemicals or vapors stimulate trigeminal and glossopharyngeal endings in the epithelial lining of the oral and nasal cavities, providing information about things like spiciness and pungency. (The latter **common chemical sense** persists even in the absence of taste buds and olfactory receptors.)

Taste Is Mediated by Receptors in Taste Buds, Innervated by Cranial Nerves VII, IX, and X

> **Key Concept**
>
> The tongue is covered by a series of papillae, some of which contain taste buds.

The surface of the tongue is covered by a series of bumps and folds (**papillae**), which are the homes of **taste buds**. **Fungiform** papillae scattered over the anterior tongue typically contain a few taste buds each. **Foliate** papillae, folds along the sides of the posterior tongue, contain dozens of taste buds each. **Circumvallate** papillae are arranged in a V-shaped row about two thirds of the way back on the tongue. They are few in number (8-9) but contain hundreds of taste buds each, accounting for about half of all the taste buds on an average tongue.

Circumvallate and most foliate papillae are innervated by the glossopharyngeal nerve (IX), fungiform and anterior foliate papillae by the facial nerve (VII). The vagus gets into the act by innervating the few taste buds farther back in the pharynx (probably more important for things like coughing when something nasty gets back there than for the perception of taste). This innervation is distinct from that taking care of touch, pain, and temperature in the mouth (Fig. 13-1).

Taste Receptor Cells Are Modified Epithelial Cells with Neuron-like Properties

> **Key Concept**
>
> Taste receptor cells utilize a variety of transduction mechanisms to detect sweet, salty, sour, and bitter stimuli.

Each taste bud (THB6 Figure 13-2, p. 325) is an encapsulated collection of **taste receptor cells**, supporting cells, and stem cells that give rise to new receptors (taste receptor cells only live for a week or two). An opening at the lingual surface of each bud lets dissolved chemicals in to contact the apical ends of the taste receptor cells.

Taste receptor cells, unlike most other receptors, are not neurons but rather are modified epithelial cells. Nevertheless, they have some very neuron-like properties:

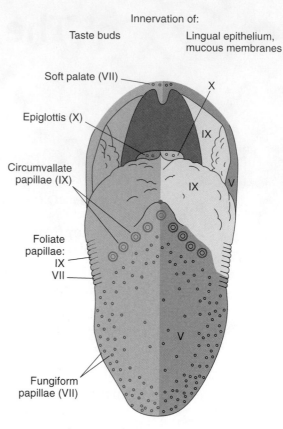

Figure 13-1   Innervation patterns of taste buds and lingual epithelium.

they make depolarizing receptor potentials (and many even make action potentials), which in turn increase the release of neurotransmitter (in this case, the principal transmitter is ATP) onto the peripheral processes of cranial nerve fibers (Fig. 13-2). Some taste receptor cells release ATP at typical chemical synapses. Others use an unusual Ca^{2+}-independent mechanism in which big voltage-gated channels open and intracellular ATP just spills out into extracellular space.

Also unlike other receptors, taste receptor cells collectively use several different transduction mechanisms. These mechanisms range from very simple ones in which the Na^+ ions in salty foods enter the cell directly through cation channels, to more complex ones in which sweet or bitter substances initiate G protein–coupled processes.

Second-Order Gustatory Neurons Are Located in the Nucleus of the Solitary Tract

Afferents that innervate taste buds reach the brainstem with the facial nerve (from the anterior two thirds of the tongue), the glossopharyngeal nerve (from the posterior third of the tongue), and the vagus nerve (from the epiglottis and esophagus). Like other visceral afferents (see Fig. 12-10) they too travel within the brainstem in the

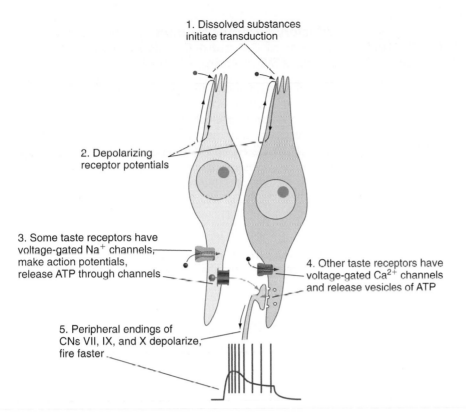

1. Dissolved substances initiate transduction

2. Depolarizing receptor potentials

3. Some taste receptors have voltage-gated Na⁺ channels, make action potentials, release ATP through channels

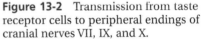

4. Other taste receptors have voltage-gated Ca^{2+} channels and release vesicles of ATP

5. Peripheral endings of CNs VII, IX, and X depolarize, fire faster

Figure 13-2 Transmission from taste receptor cells to peripheral endings of cranial nerves VII, IX, and X.

solitary tract and end in the **nucleus of the solitary tract**, mostly in more rostral portions (Fig. 13-3).

Gustatory neurons in the nucleus of the solitary tract participate in feeding (e.g., salivating, swallowing) and protective activities (e.g., coughing). They also convey information to the thalamus and from there to gustatory cortex in the insula (conscious awareness of taste) and indirectly to the hypothalamus and amygdala (pleasantness or unpleasantness of taste). Unlike other ascending sensory pathways to the thalamus, the gustatory pathway is uncrossed.

Information about Taste Is Coded, in Part, by the Pattern of Activity in Populations of Neurons

We usually think of sensory receptors as being good at signaling the location of a stimulus, but this doesn't work for taste buds. When we eat or drink, dissolved chemicals and vapors get distributed widely in the mouth and nose, so the stimulated taste buds and olfactory receptors can't provide accurate information about the location of the stimulus; we use somatosensory cues instead to decide this. The major task of the gustatory and olfactory systems is to analyze the composition of mixtures of potentially thousands of chemicals. In principle, we could do this by having one kind of taste receptor specifically tuned to the taste of radishes, another to rutabagas, etc., but this would require an unwieldy number of receptor types. So instead we compare the levels of activity in populations of receptors, each population responsive to more than one kind of chemical. This is a lot like comparing the levels of activity in just three kinds of cones (see Chapter 17) to identify hundreds of colors.

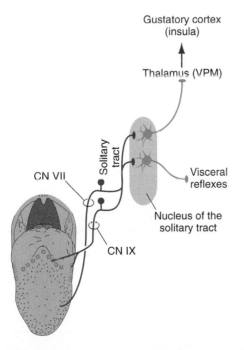

Gustatory cortex (insula)

Thalamus (VPM)

Solitary tract

CN VII

Visceral reflexes

Nucleus of the solitary tract

CN IX

Figure 13-3 CNS taste connections. (Further connections with the hypothalamus and amygdala not indicated.)

Olfaction Is Mediated by Receptors That Project Directly to the Telencephalon

Key Concept

The axons of olfactory receptor neurons form CN I.

The olfactory pathway begins with bipolar receptor cells whose chemosensitive processes project into the layer of mucus covering the **olfactory epithelium**. These are long receptors, and the same receptor cells have thin axons (Fig. 13-4) that pass through the ethmoid bone as the **olfactory nerve** (**CN I**) and end in the **olfactory bulb**. Olfactory receptors are therefore highly unusual in having processes exposed to the outside world and in having axons that project directly to the telencephalon. They are also unusual in being neurons that are continuously replaced throughout life.

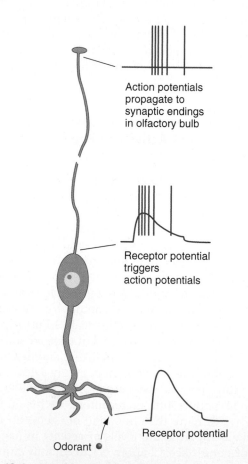

Figure 13-4 Signaling by olfactory receptors.

Olfactory Receptor Neurons Utilize a Large Number of G Protein–Coupled Receptors to Detect a Wide Range of Odors

The olfactory system, like the gustatory system, compares the levels of activity in populations of receptors, each population responsive to more than one kind of chemical. We can discriminate many more kinds of odors than tastes, and corresponding to this there are numerous kinds of olfactory receptors. However, all of them use closely related receptor proteins and the same G protein–coupled transduction mechanism (THB6 Figure 13-12, p. 334).

Olfactory Information Bypasses the Thalamus on Its Way to the Cerebral Cortex

Key Concepts

The olfactory nerve terminates in the olfactory bulb.
The olfactory bulb projects to olfactory cortex.
Olfactory information reaches other cortical areas both directly and via the thalamus.

The olfactory system continues to break the rules by projecting to cerebral cortex without first relaying in the thalamus (Fig. 13-5). The fibers of the **olfactory tract**, which arises in the olfactory bulb, end in anterior temporal cortex (**piriform cortex** and nearby areas), as well as in the **amygdala** and in areas at the base of the brain (**anterior perforated substance**). Piriform and nearby cortex, however, is not **neocortex** like the cortex that covers most of the cerebral hemispheres (see Chapter 22); it has a simpler structure and is referred to as **paleocortex**. There is an additional olfactory area in neocortex, in the orbital cortex of the frontal lobe, where olfactory information converges with projections from gustatory cortex. In this case the rules are followed more

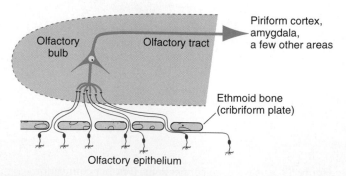

Figure 13-5 Olfactory CNS connections.

closely: Information from piriform cortex reaches the orbital olfactory/gustatory area via a relay in the dorsomedial nucleus of the thalamus (as well as via direct projections). As in the case of gustatory pathways, all of these olfactory connections are mostly uncrossed.

Conductive and Sensorineural Problems Can Affect Olfactory Function

Olfaction can be impaired both by processes that prevent things from reaching olfactory receptors (**conductive deficit**) and by damage in the nervous system (**sensorineural** deficit). We have probably all experienced conductive deficits during the stuffiness of colds or allergic conditions. Sensorineural deficits are a common result of head trauma, for example because of a shear injury to olfactory nerve fibers as they pass through the ethmoid bone. Some degenerative conditions, notably Parkinson's and Alzheimer's diseases, can also affect the olfactory system. A selective sensorineural olfactory deficit does not involve the common chemical sense, so sensitivity to things like menthol and ammonia may be unaffected. Hence, it is important to use things like coffee, vanilla, or floral extracts to test olfaction.

Multiple Flavor-Related Signals Converge in Orbital Cortex

All the different factors that determine how we experience a food or beverage—its appearance, aromas, basic taste, texture, temperature—come together in orbital cortex, by way of projections from visual, olfactory, gustatory, and somatosensory cortical areas (THB6 Figure 13-21, p. 339). The same orbital area gets inputs from limbic structures like the amygdala, reflecting the influence of hunger and cravings on how things taste.

Study Questions

1. A 39-year-old handball player tripped and fell while backpedaling, striking the back of his head hard on the floor. The next day he noticed that food no longer seemed to have much taste. Being a curious sort he began to experiment on himself, noting that he had no trouble perceiving the texture or temperature of food. Cola and tonic water tasted almost normal, and he could easily taste a few crystals of salt he placed on his tongue. A household cleaning solution (which he had forgotten he owned) smelled sharp and unpleasant. The most likely cause of this condition was
   a. avulsion of the lingual nerves.
   b. medullary hemorrhage affecting the solitary tracts.
   c. tearing of olfactory nerve fibers.
   d. uncal herniation.
2. The axons in the solitary tract
   a. are central branches of facial, glossopharyngeal, and hypoglossal fibers.
   b. convey gustatory and olfactory chemosensory information.
   c. mostly terminate in nucleus ambiguus.
   d. serve as the afferent limb of a variety of reflexes, including those that modulate cardiac and respiratory function.
3. Olfactory inputs reach olfactory cortex (piriform cortex) via
   a. olfactory receptors that synapse on ganglion cells in the olfactory nerve; these ganglion cells project to the olfactory bulb, whose cells in turn project to olfactory cortex.
   b. olfactory receptors whose axons enter the olfactory bulb directly; neurons of the olfactory bulb then project through the olfactory tract to olfactory cortex.
   c. olfactory receptors that project to the olfactory bulb, which in turn projects to olfactory cortex via a thalamic relay in the anterior geniculate nucleus.
   d. olfactory receptors that are hollow and actually duct the chemical odorants into the olfactory bulb, where a little fan blows them onward toward the cortex.

4. The taste buds of fungiform papillae (the ones near the front of the tongue) are innervated primarily by cranial nerve
   a. V
   b. VII
   c. IX
   d. X
   e. XII
5. Taste and olfactory receptor cells are similar in that both
   a. use only G protein–coupled transduction mechanisms.
   b. respond to a very narrowly tuned range of chemicals.
   c. regularly die and are replaced.
   d. have long axons that convey action potentials to the CNS.

Hearing and Balance: The Eighth Cranial Nerve

14

The eighth nerve is the nerve of hearing and equilibrium. All of its receptive functions are accomplished by variations on a common theme; the different sensory information carried by different fibers in the nerve is simply the result of slight differences in the mechanical arrangement of receptors and accessory structures.

Auditory and Vestibular Receptor Cells Are Located in the Walls of the Membranous Labyrinth

> **Key Concept**
>
> The membranous labyrinth is suspended within the bony labyrinth, a cavity in the temporal bone.

Eighth nerve fibers innervate special receptors called **hair cells**, located in an elaborate end organ called the **labyrinth** (THB6 Figures 14-1 and 14-2, pp. 343 and 344). The labyrinth is two series of twisted tubes (hence the name labyrinth), one suspended inside the other (THB6 Figure 14-3, p. 345). The outer tube, the **bony labyrinth**, is a continuous channel in the temporal bone. The **bony cochlea** is located anteriorly, the **bony semicircular canals** posteriorly, and the **vestibule** between the two. The inner tube (so to speak), the **membranous labyrinth**, is a second continuous tube suspended within the bony labyrinth; as explained a little later, the mechanical arrangement of the cochlear suspension is crucial to its function. The membranous labyrinth generally parallels portions of the bony labyrinth (i.e., there are **cochlear** and **semicircular ducts**), except that the vestibule contains two parts of the membranous labyrinth—the **utricle** and the **saccule**.

Endolymph Is Actively Secreted, Circulates through the Membranous Labyrinth, and Is Reabsorbed

The bony labyrinth is filled with **perilymph**, which is more or less equivalent to cerebrospinal fluid and actually communicates with subarachnoid CSF. The membranous labyrinth, in contrast, is filled with **endolymph**, whose ionic composition more closely resembles that inside a cell (i.e., high $[K^+]$, low $[Na^+]$). Endolymph is secreted by specialized cells in the walls of the membranous labyrinth, circulates through it, and is reabsorbed.

Auditory and Vestibular Receptors Are Hair Cells

> **Key Concepts**
>
> Hair cells have mechanosensitive transduction channels.
> Subtle differences in the physical arrangements of hair cells determine the stimuli to which they are most sensitive.

Hair cells, the characteristic receptor cells of the labyrinth, have a graduated array of specialized microvilli (**stereocilia**) and sometimes one true cilium (the **kinocilium**) on their apical surfaces. Each stereocilium is attached to its next tallest neighbor by a filamentous **tip link** protein, connected at one or both ends to a cation channel. The sensory hairs of the hair cells poke through the wall of the membranous labyrinth and are typically inserted into a mass of gelatinous material (Fig. 14-1). Movement of a hair bundle relative to the gelatinous material causes a depolarizing or a hyperpolarizing receptor potential, depending on the direction of deflection. Deflecting the hair bundle toward the tallest stereocilia stretches the tip links, opens the cation channels,

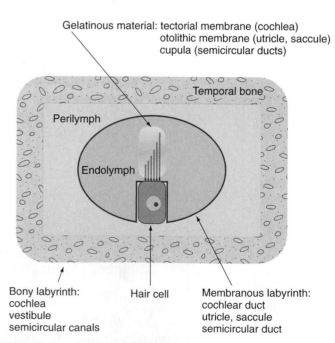

Gelatinous material: tectorial membrane (cochlea)
otolithic membrane (utricle, saccule)
cupula (semicircular ducts)

Temporal bone

Perilymph

Endolymph

Bony labyrinth:
cochlea
vestibule
semicircular canals

Hair cell

Membranous labyrinth:
cochlear duct
utricle, saccule
semicircular duct

Figure 14-1 Overview of the labyrinth; all the terms are explained at various places in this chapter. The wall of the membranous labyrinth is drawn in red to indicate that it's a diffusion barrier between perilymph and endolymph. Even though hair cells (in histological sections) seem to be contained within the membranous labyrinth, they are actually bathed mostly in perilymph.

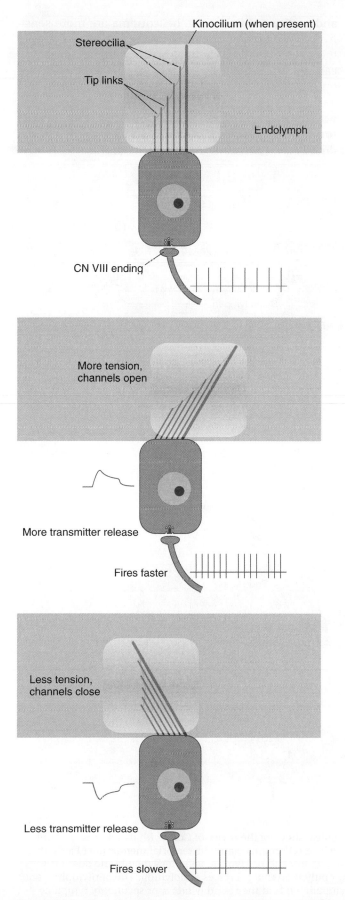

Figure 14-2 Transduction by hair cells, and transmission to eighth nerve fibers.

and depolarizes the hair cell; deflecting in the opposite direction lets the tip links relax, and some channels that were open at rest close. This in turn causes an increase or a decrease in the release of an excitatory transmitter (probably glutamate), and a consequent increase or decrease in the firing rate of any eighth nerve fiber that innervates the hair cell (Fig. 14-2). The way in which the gelatinous material is arranged within the labyrinth plays a major role in determining the kind of mechanical stimulus to which a particular region of the labyrinth responds best.

The Cochlear Division of the Eighth Nerve Conveys Information about Sound

The auditory apparatus has three general areas—the **outer**, **middle**, and **inner ears**. The outer and middle ears (separated from each other by the **tympanic membrane**) are air-filled cavities in or leading into the temporal bone; the inner ear is the fluid-filled labyrinth.

The Outer and Middle Ears Convey Airborne Vibrations to the Fluid-Filled Inner Ear

Sound vibrations are funneled through the outer ear and vibrate the tympanic membrane. This in turn vibrates the **malleus**, **incus**, and **stapes** (the middle ear **ossicles**), and the stapes footplate vibrates the perilymph of the inner ear through the **oval window**. (Inward pushes and outward pulls of the stapes are accommodated by outward and inward bulges of the **round window membrane**.) This elaborate mechanism is necessary because sound does not cross an air-water interface very well, and there is essentially an air-water interface between the outside world and the perilymph of the cochlea. The slight mechanical advantage of the middle ear ossicles, together with the much larger area of the tympanic membrane relative to the oval window, results in a much greater force per unit area at the oval window than at the tympanic membrane.

The Cochlea Is the Auditory Part of the Labyrinth

> **Key Concept**
>
> Traveling waves in the basilar membrane stimulate hair cells in the organ of Corti, in locations that depend on sound frequency.

The cochlear duct is stretched as a partition across the cochlear part of the bony labyrinth. The partition is complete except for a small hole at the apex of the cochlea (the **helicotrema**) at which two otherwise separate perilymphatic spaces communicate with each other. Therefore when the stapes moves inward and outward, part of the resulting perilymph movement causes a **traveling wave** of deformation that moves along the cochlear duct. The deformation reaches a maximum amplitude at a site that depends on the frequency of the stapes vibration (Fig. 14-3); portions of the cochlear duct closer to the oval window are more sensitive to higher frequencies, and portions closer to the helicotrema are more sensitive to lower frequencies. This is, at least to a great extent, the result of gradual changes in the width and mechanical properties of the **basilar membrane**, which forms one wall of the cochlear duct. Cochlear hair cells are located in the **organ of Corti** (on the basilar membrane), with their sensory hairs embedded in the gelatinous **tectorial membrane** (Fig. 14-4). Deformation of the cochlear duct causes differential movement of the basilar and tec-

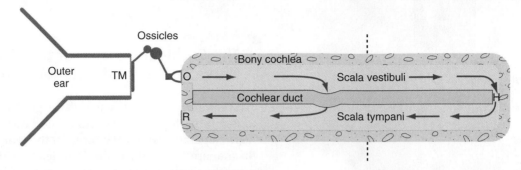

Figure 14-3   Outer, middle, and inner ear, shown schematically as though the cochlea had been uncoiled. Vibrations transmitted through the tympanic membrane (TM), middle ear ossicles, and oval window (O) reach the perilymph of the inner ear. Very low frequencies and static pressure changes move perilymph through the helicotrema (H), but audible frequencies deform the cochlear duct. The *dashed line* indicates the plane of section in Fig. 14-4. *R*, Round window membrane.

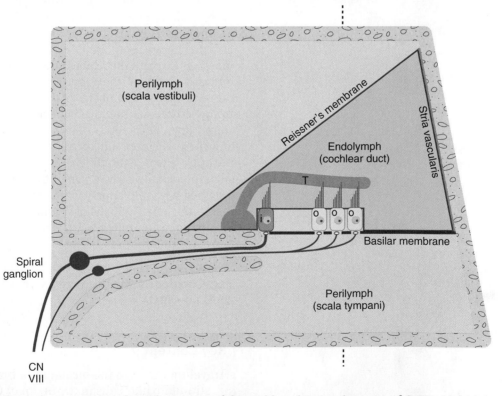

Figure 14-4   A schematic cross section through one turn of the cochlea, showing the organ of Corti with its inner (i) and outer (o) hair cells. The tallest stereocilia of at least the outer hair cells are inserted in the gelatinous tectorial membrane (T). All three walls of the cochlear duct contain a diffusion barrier separating endolymph and perilymph. Reissner's membrane does little more than this, but the stria vascularis is specialized as a secretory epithelium that produces endolymph. The perilymph of scala vestibuli (open to the vestibule) is continuous with that of scala tympani (ends at the round window, or secondary tympanic membrane) at the helicotrema. The *dashed line* indicates the plane of section in Fig. 14-3.

torial membranes and this deflects the sensory hairs, which in turn causes either a depolarizing or a hyperpolarizing receptor potential in the hair cells (depending on the direction of deflection).

Inner Hair Cells Are Sensory Cells; Outer Hair Cells Are Amplifiers

There are two populations of cochlear hair cells all along the basilar membrane. **Inner hair cells** are closer to the center of the cochlea, less numerous, but heavily innervated by eighth nerve fibers; they are the principal source of the sound information conveyed by the eighth nerve. **Outer hair cells** are more numerous but sparsely innervated. The main job of the outer hair cells is not to transmit auditory information to eighth nerve fibers, but rather to lengthen and shorten very rapidly in response to the receptor potentials they produce when the basilar membrane vibrates. This movement in turn enhances the responses of nearby inner hair cells, making a major contribution to their sensitivity and frequency selectivity.

The basilar membrane vibrations caused by outer hair cell movement are transmitted back along the middle ear ossicles and reach the tympanic membrane, turning it, in effect, into a tiny loudspeaker. The resulting

otoacoustic emissions can be detected by a sensitive microphone in the ear canal, forming the basis of a clinical test of hair cell function.

Auditory Information Is Distributed Bilaterally in the CNS

We use our ears not only to identify sounds, but also to localize them in space. This localization is achieved by comparing time and intensity differences between the sounds arriving at our two ears, and the comparison begins early in the CNS. Cochlear nerve fibers end ipsilaterally in the **cochlear nuclei** at the pontomedullary junction. The cochlear nuclei then project bilaterally in the brainstem, so at all levels rostral to the cochlear nuclei each ear is represented bilaterally (Fig. 14-5) and unilateral damage does not cause deafness of either ear. Rostral to the cochlear nuclei, the auditory pathway on each side is concerned not so much with one ear as with information from both ears relevant to the contralateral half of the auditory world.

Successively more rostral stages in the auditory pathway (THB6 Figure 14-18, p. 359) include the **superior olivary nucleus** (crossing fibers reach it through the **trapezoid body**); **inferior colliculus** (by way of the **lateral lemniscus**); **medial geniculate nucleus** of the

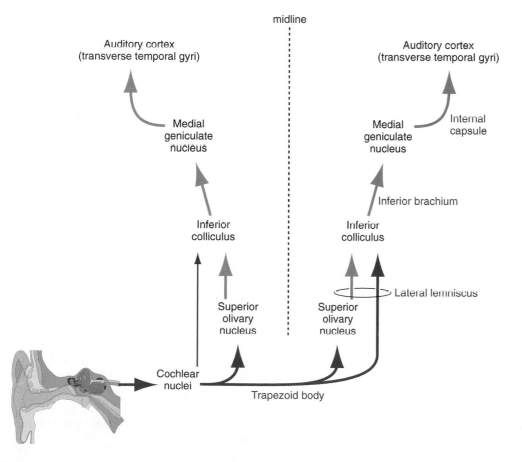

Figure 14-5 The CNS auditory pathway. Projections representing just one ear are shown in blue, those representing both ears in green.

thalamus (by way of the **brachium of the inferior colliculus**, or **inferior brachium**); and **auditory cortex** (transverse temporal gyri on the superior surface of the temporal lobe).

Activity in the Ascending Auditory Pathway Generates Electrical Signals That Can Be Measured from the Scalp

It takes time for electrical activity to move from the cochlea, along the eighth nerve, and then from one brainstem stop to the next. One consequence is that signal-averaging computers can be used to record (from the scalp) a series of waves with predictable latencies in response to repeated auditory stimuli like clicks (THB6 Figure 14-20, p. 361). Changes in the latencies of these waves, or the disappearance of some of them, can be used to help localize neural damage.

Efferents Control the Sensitivity of the Cochlea

> **Key Concepts**
>
> Middle ear muscles contract in response to loud sounds.
> Different sets of efferents control outer hair cells and the afferent endings on inner hair cells.

The CNS controls the sensitivity of the cochlea in multiple ways, from regulating the stiffness of the middle ear ossicular chain to regulating hair cell function.

Two small muscles—the **stapedius**, attached to the stapes, and the **tensor tympani**, attached to the malleus—affect middle ear function by tugging on ossicles and decreasing their ability to transmit vibrations. The tensor tympani is only activated by very loud sounds, and its function is unclear. However, the stapedius is activated bilaterally in response to loud sounds near the upper end of the physiological range of intensities. Stapedial contraction makes the tympanic membrane harder to vibrate, so more sound gets reflected from it. Hence measuring the amount of a test sound reflected from one tympanic membrane provides an indirect measure of stapedius contraction on that side. The circuitry of the **acoustic (stapedius) reflex** involves both the seventh and eighth nerves, as well some of their central connections (Fig. 14-6), so this forms the basis of a useful clinical test.

Still another set of neurons in the superior olivary nucleus project not into the ascending auditory pathway, but instead to the organ of Corti (THB6 Figure 14-21, p. 362). Some suppress the contractility of outer hair cells, possibly helping to filter out high-frequency noise;

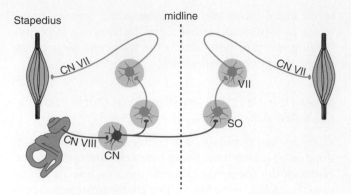

Figure 14-6 Acoustic (stapedius) reflex connections. *CN*, Cochlear nuclei; *SO*, superior olivary nucleus; *VII*, facial motor nucleus.

others regulate transmission from inner hair cells to eighth nerve fibers.

Conductive and Sensorineural Problems Can Affect Hearing

Just as in the case of olfaction, hearing can be impaired by two general kinds of processes: those that impair the ability of air-borne vibrations to reach the organ of Corti (**conductive hearing loss**) and those that impair the ability of hair cells or the cochlear nerve to respond (**sensorineural hearing loss**). Conductive hearing loss (e.g., from a middle ear infection) affects only the ability to hear sounds delivered by air; it has no effect on the threshold for vibrations delivered by a probe pressed against the skull. So impaired hearing in one ear measured by **air conduction**, but normal hearing by **bone conduction**, indicates a conductive hearing loss in that ear. In contrast, sensorineural damage (e.g., from noise exposure or an eighth nerve tumor) results in impaired hearing no matter what route is used to deliver vibrations.

The Vestibular Division of the Eighth Nerve Conveys Information about Linear and Angular Acceleration of the Head

The vestibular parts of the labyrinth use basically the same kind of hair cell-gelatinous material mechanism as the organ of Corti. However, these parts of the membranous labyrinth are suspended inside the bony labyrinth, surrounded by perilymph, so sound vibrations are distributed uniformly around them and have no effect. Instead, different specializations of the gelatinous material and its coupling to hair cells make the utricle and saccule sensitive to linear acceleration and the semicircular ducts to angular acceleration.

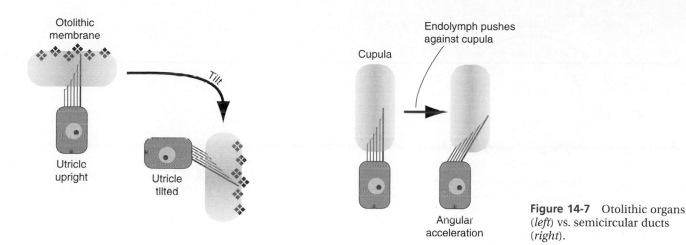

Figure 14-7 Otolithic organs (*left*) vs. semicircular ducts (*right*).

Receptors in the Utricle and Saccule Detect Linear Acceleration and Position of the Head

The utricle and saccule each contains a flattened patch of hair cells (a **macula**) overlain by a layer of gelatinous material containing crystals of calcium carbonate (hence called an **otolithic membrane**, or a "membrane full of ear stones"). The otolithic membrane is denser than endolymph and so tries to move through it in response to gravity or other linear accelerations (Fig. 14-7). This in turn deflects the hair bundles inserted into the otolithic membrane and elicits depolarizing or hyperpolarizing receptor potentials. The utricular macula is oriented in a mostly horizontal plane (i.e., stereocilia pointing toward the sky), the saccular macula in a mostly vertical plane. Hence, the utricle is most sensitive to tilts beginning from a head-upright position, the saccule to tilts beginning from a head-sideways position. In response to linear acceleration in its plane, an otolithic membrane lags behind because of inertia. As a result, the utricle also responds to acceleration in horizontal planes (front-back, side to side), and the saccule to acceleration in vertical planes (front-back, up-down).

Receptors in the Semicircular Ducts Detect Angular Acceleration of the Head

Key Concept

Conditions that make the cupula sensitive to gravity cause nystagmus and illusions of movement.

The semicircular ducts use a different mechanism. Each contains a dilatation called an **ampulla**, in which the hair cells reside as part of a ridge called a **crista**. The hair bundles are inserted into a gelatinous diaphragm called a **cupula**. Movement of the endolymph within a semicircular duct would therefore distort the cupula and deflect the hair bundles (see Fig. 14-7).

The most effective stimulus for causing such movement is angular acceleration in the plane of a given canal (like a wheel on an axle). For example, at the beginning of rotation the endolymph lags behind because of inertia and pushes the cupula in the opposite direction. After a few seconds the endolymph catches up, and at the end of rotation it continues to move, again because of inertia, and pushes the cupula in the direction of the previous rotation (Fig. 14-8). The cupula normally has the same density as endolymph, so gravity has no effect on it. Processes that change the relative densities of cupula and endolymph can make one or more semicircular ducts gravity-sensitive, so certain head positions can fool the brain into thinking there's some angular acceleration taking place. **Vertigo** results.

There are three semicircular canals and ducts on each side, in three orthogonal planes (Fig. 14-9). Roughly speaking, one is horizontal, one extends anteriorly at 45° to the sagittal plane, and one extends posteriorly at 45° to the sagittal plane. Hence, angular acceleration in any plane can be detected by each set of semicircular ducts.

Vestibular Primary Afferents Project to the Vestibular Nuclei and the Cerebellum

Vestibular primary afferents mostly end in the **vestibular nuclei**, although some reach the cerebellum directly (the only primary afferents that get to the cerebellum, primarily to the **flocculonodular lobe**).

The Vestibular Nuclei Project to the Spinal Cord, Cerebellum, and Nuclei of Cranial Nerves III, IV, and VI

Key Concept

Vestibulospinal fibers influence antigravity muscles and neck muscles.

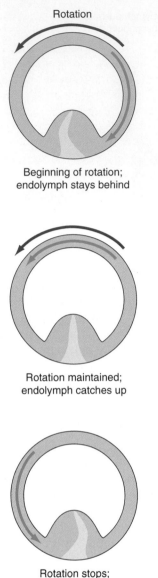

Rotation

Beginning of rotation;
endolymph stays behind

Rotation maintained;
endolymph catches up

Rotation stops;
endolymph keeps going

Figure 14-8   Semicircular ducts and angular acceleration.

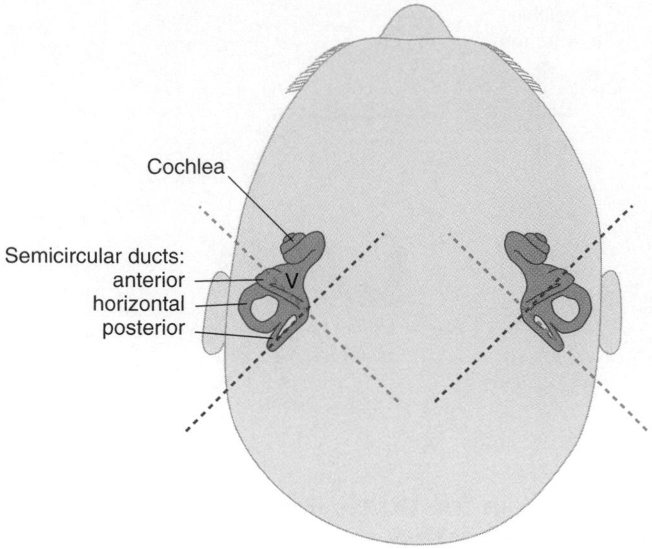

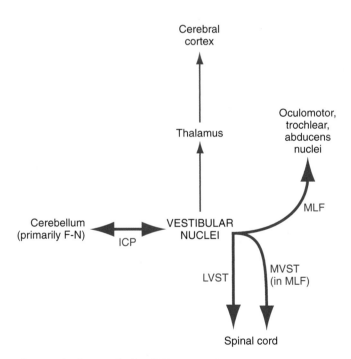

Figure 14-9   Orientation of the labyrinth, as seen from above (not to scale). *V*, Vestibule.

Figure 14-10   Vestibular CNS connections.
F-N, Flocculonodular lobe; *ICP*, inferior cerebellar peduncle; *LVST*, lateral vestibulospinal tract; *MLF*, medial longitudinal fasciculus; *MVST*, medial vestibulospinal tract.

Outputs from the vestibular nuclei go mostly to places that make sense from a functional point of view (Fig. 14-10; see THB6 Figure 14-29, p. 369). There is a vestibular projection through the thalamus to the cerebral cortex (insula and parietal lobe), but for the most part vestibular projections influence posture and eye movements.

We make postural adjustments in response to vestibular stimuli like tilts, accelerations, and rotations. Corresponding to this, there are two vestibulospinal tracts. The medial vestibular nucleus projects a bilateral **medial vestibulospinal tract** to the cervical spinal cord through the MLF. The lateral vestibular nucleus sends the uncrossed **lateral vestibulospinal tract** to all cord levels. We use the medial vestibulospinal tract to coordinate head and eye

movements and the lateral vestibulospinal tract to make postural adjustments in antigravity muscles.

The Vestibular Nuclei Participate in the Vestibulo-ocular Reflex

We can keep our eyes pointed at something even if we're moving around. That is, a head movement of 5° to the

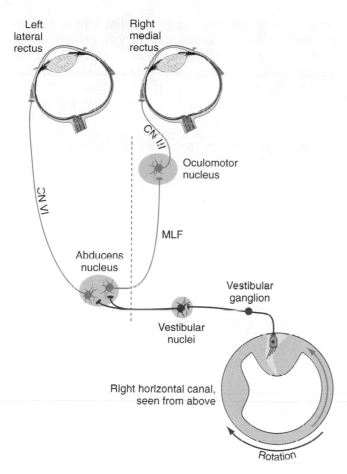

Figure 14-11 Vestibulo-ocular reflex connections.

left can be automatically nulled by a conjugate eye movement of 5° to the right. For slow head movements with your eyes open, this is partly a visual tracking movement, but you can do it even in the dark, and you can do it while your head is moving faster than visual tracking movements can work. The additional basis for these compensatory eye movements is the **vestibulo-ocular reflex**, a simple three-neuron reflex arc (Fig. 14-11). Vestibular primary afferents project to the vestibular nuclei, which then project (mostly, but not entirely, through the MLF) to the nuclei of III, IV, and VI.

Nystagmus Can Be Physiological or Pathological

Consider in a little more detail what would happen at the beginning of rotation to your left in the dark. At first, the vestibulo-ocular reflex would move your eyes to the right, the appropriate movement to keep the direction in which your eyes are pointed from changing (i.e., to keep your gaze from shifting). However, there is obviously a limit to how far your eyes can rotate in their sockets, and if you continue to spin around these compensatory movements are periodically interrupted by fast "reset" movements in the opposite direction. The

combined back-and-forth movement is called **nystagmus**, and it gets named for the direction of the fast component. Hence, at the beginning of rotation to the left there would be nystagmus to the left ("left-beating nystagmus"). If rotation is maintained in the dark, the vestibular stimulus loses its effectiveness (see Fig. 14-8) and the **rotatory** nystagmus ceases. Right after a rotation ends, the direction of cupula deflection is the opposite of that at the beginning of rotation (see Fig. 14-8), and so there is **postrotatory** nystagmus in the opposite direction.

The same nystagmus can be elicited by moving a repetitive visual stimulus in front of someone. In this case it is called **optokinetic** nystagmus. The nystagmus at the beginning of rotation with the lights on is a combination of rotatory and optokinetic nystagmus (both in the same direction because both are reflex attempts to maintain visual stability). If the rotation continues with the lights on, optokinetic nystagmus may persist.

Stimulating a single horizontal semicircular canal is sufficient to cause nystagmus, and this can be done **calorically** using warm or cool water. With the head tilted back so that the horizontal canal is in an approximately vertical plane, the temperature change causes endolymphatic convection currents that mimic those caused by angular acceleration. Cool water in one ear causes nystagmus with its fast phase to the opposite side, and warm water causes nystagmus with its fast phase to the same side (THB6 Figure 14-33, p. 373).

Position Sense Is Mediated by the Vestibular, Proprioceptive, and Visual Systems Acting Together

The vestibular system plays a major role, but not the only role, in our ability to sense and maintain our orientation with respect to gravity, as well as in our ability to maintain visual fixation while we move. Contrary to what you might think, the thing it's most indispensable for is helping with eye movements. People with bilateral vestibular loss recover to a point where their sense of orientation is pretty good, but they continue to have trouble maintaining gaze unless they move relatively slowly.

We actually use three different sensory systems to tell us about position and movement—vestibular, visual, and somatosensory (especially neck receptors). People can do pretty well with only two of these systems, and that's the basis for compensation after loss of vestibular function. If two of the three systems aren't working, we have a lot of trouble. For example, someone with no vestibular function or deficient somatosensory function would be very disabled in the dark. The three systems can interact in sometimes surprising ways: Visual-vestibular conflicts can cause striking illusions of movement; neck dysfunction can cause vertigo.

Information from these three systems needs to be integrated at an early stage. As one example, the semicircular canals can only signal maintained rotation for a little while, but the postural adjustments need to be maintained or you fall down. As a second example, if you were resting your head on your desk and your chair started to slide out, you'd probably make postural adjustments even though there had been no vestibular input. This integration starts to happen at the level of the vestibular nuclei, which up until now we have pretended received only vestibular and cerebellar inputs. In fact, the same cells receive somatosensory and visual inputs. In the first example, visual inputs to the vestibular nuclei cause continued nystagmus (called optokinetic nystagmus in this case because it is maintained by moving visual stimuli) and postural adjustments just as the original vestibular signal did. In the second example, the neck-vestibular mismatch would cause a vestibulospinal output.

Study Questions

1. A patient was observed to have no acoustic (stapedius) reflex in her left ear in response to loud sounds in either ear. However, loud sounds in either ear caused an acoustic reflex in her right ear. The most likely site of damage was her
    a. left facial nerve.
    b. right facial nerve.
    c. left trigeminal nerve.
    d. right trigeminal nerve.
    e. left eighth nerve.
    f. right eighth nerve.

2. A patient complained of trouble hearing with his right ear. You find that if you hold a vibrating tuning fork by his right ear until he can no longer hear it, he can hear it again if you move it to his left ear or press it against either mastoid process. The most likely cause of his hearing problem is
    a. bony growths that impede vibrations of the right middle ear bones.
    b. noise-induced loss of hair cells from the right cochlea.
    c. an acoustic neuroma that compromises the right eighth nerve.
    d. damage to the right lateral lemniscus.
    e. damage to the left lateral lemniscus.

3. The membranous labyrinth
    a. is filled with perilymph.
    b. includes the vestibule.
    c. includes the saccule.
    d. a and c.
    e. none of the above.

4. Hair cells that synapse on eighth nerve fibers
    a. have sensory hairs bathed in endolymph.
    b. can produce both hyperpolarizing and depolarizing receptor potentials, depending on the direction in which their hair bundles are deflected.
    c. all work by having fluid currents deflect their hair bundles.
    d. a and b.
    e. all of the above.

5. The most important factor in efficient transfer of sound energy into the inner ear is
    a. the relative sizes of the tympanic membrane and the oval window.
    b. the mechanical advantage provided by the middle ear ossicles.
    c. funneling of sound by the outer ear.
    d. the ionic composition of perilymph, which allows sound to cross an air-perilymph interface with great efficiency.

6. Endolymph
    a. fills the utricle.
    b. bathes the synapses between hair cells and eighth nerve fibers.
    c. has a sodium concentration similar to that of cerebrospinal fluid.
    d. flows through the helicotrema.

7. Outer hair cells
    a. are found exclusively near the apex of the cochlea, accounting for the fact that the apex of the cochlea is most sensitive to high frequencies.
    b. are found exclusively near the apex of the cochlea, accounting for the fact that the apex of the cochlea is most sensitive to low frequencies.
    c. are found at all levels of the cochlea; the increased sensitivity of the apex of the cochlea to high frequencies is caused by other factors.
    d. are found at all levels of the cochlea; the increased sensitivity of the apex of the cochlea to low frequencies is caused by other factors.

8. The gelatinous substance into which cochlear hair bundles are inserted is called the
    a. tectorial membrane.
    b. otolithic membrane.
    c. cupula.
    d. basilar membrane.

9. Both ears are represented in all of the following nuclei *except* the
    a. superior olivary nucleus.
    b. inferior colliculus.
    c. cochlear nuclei.
    d. medial geniculate nucleus.
    e. Both ears are represented in all of these nuclei.

10. Primary auditory cortex is located in the
    a. parietal lobe, just posterior to the postcentral gyrus.
    b. lateral surface of the occipital lobe.
    c. transverse temporal gyri.
    d. inferior temporal gyrus.
    e. middle frontal gyrus.

11. Keeping your head tilted forward 15° would most effectively stimulate hair cells in the
    a. utricle.
    b. saccule.
    c. semicircular ducts.

Study Questions—Cont'd

12. Interactions among the vestibular, visual and somatosensory systems first occur in the
    a. parietal lobe.
    b. vestibular nuclei.
    c. spinal cord.
    d. occipital lobe.
    e. temporal lobe.

13. A mad neuroanatomist built an apparatus for demonstrating the activity of the vestibular system and somehow persuaded a local goldfish trainer to try it out. The goldfish trainer crawled into a horizontal tube, lay down on his back, and rested his head on a 30° wedge so that his head was tilted upward. The neuroanatomist turned out the lights and turned on a motor that spun the tube on its long axis, to the goldfish trainer's right, and then left the room for a while. Electrical recordings of the goldfish trainer's eye movements would have shown nystagmus
    a. to the left (fast phase) for several seconds, then a period of no nystagmus, then nystagmus to the right when the rotation stopped.
    b. to the left for the duration of the rotation, then nystagmus to the right when the rotation stopped.
    c. to the right for several seconds, then a period of no nystagmus, then nystagmus to the left when the rotation stopped.
    d. to the right for the duration of the rotation, then nystagmus to the left when the rotation stopped.
    e. to the left throughout the rotation, and for several seconds after the rotation stopped.

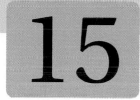

Brainstem Summary

The previous four chapters presented various aspects of the brainstem and its cranial nerves bit by bit. This chapter summarizes the major points, using as a vehicle the same series of drawings of brainstem sections used in Chapter 11, but with additional structures and brief descriptions added. A few of the structures (e.g., substantia nigra) are dealt with more fully in later chapters.

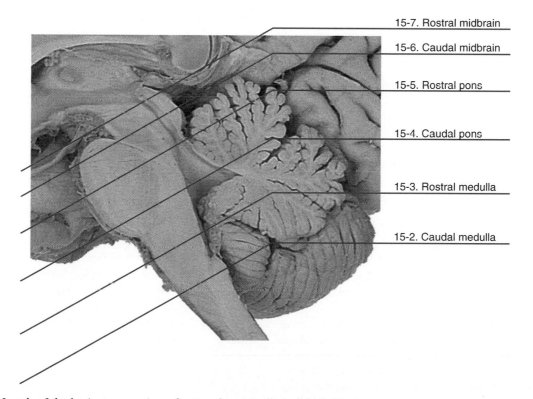

15-7. Rostral midbrain

15-6. Caudal midbrain

15-5. Rostral pons

15-4. Caudal pons

15-3. Rostral medulla

15-2. Caudal medulla

Figure 15-1 Levels of the brainstem sections shown schematically in this chapter.

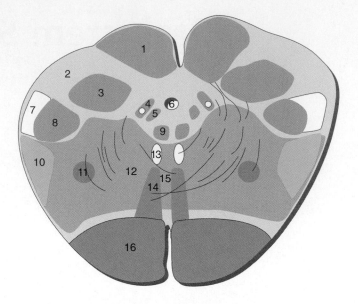

Figure 15-2   Caudal medulla.

Caudal Medulla

1. *Nucleus gracilis.* Second-order somatosensory neurons whose axons cross at this level to form the leg portion of the medial lemniscus.

2. *Fasciculus cuneatus.* Uncrossed branches of primary afferents, carrying tactile and proprioceptive information from the arm.

3. *Nucleus cuneatus.* Second-order somatosensory neurons whose axons cross at this level to form the arm portion of the medial lemniscus.

4. *Nucleus of the solitary tract,* surrounding the solitary tract. This is much like a posterior column system for information from viscera and taste buds: Central branches of afferents from cranial nerves VII, IX, and X travel through the tract to reach the nucleus. Only information from viscera reaches this caudal level.

5. *Dorsal motor nucleus of the vagus.* Preganglionic parasympathetic neurons for thoracic and abdominal viscera.

6. *Central canal.* Continuous rostrally with the fourth ventricle and caudally with the central canal of the spinal cord.

7. *Spinal trigeminal tract.* Primary afferents from the ipsilateral side of the face, at this caudal level conveying information about pain and temperature.

8. *Spinal trigeminal nucleus.* At this caudal level, second-order pain and temperature neurons whose axons cross the midline and join the anterolateral pathway. Trigeminal pain and temperature afferents from the ipsilateral face reach the nucleus via the spinal trigeminal tract.

9. *Hypoglossal nucleus.* Lower motor neurons for ipsilateral tongue muscles.

10. *Anterolateral pathway.* Mostly crossed fibers of second-order spinal neurons conveying pain and temperature information to the thalamus (spinothalamic tract), reticular formation, and midbrain.

11. *Location of nucleus ambiguus.* Lower motor neurons for laryngeal and pharyngeal muscles (also contains preganglionic parasympathetic neurons for the heart).

12. *Reticular formation.*

13. *Medial longitudinal fasciculus (MLF).* At this level, the fibers of the medial vestibulospinal tract.

14. *Medial lemniscus,* the principal ascending pathway for tactile and proprioceptive information. Originates in the contralateral posterior column nuclei and terminates in the thalamus (VPL).

15. *Raphe nuclei.* Widely projecting serotonergic neurons that collectively blanket the CNS. Those in caudal brainstem levels like this project mainly to the spinal cord.

16. *Pyramid.* Corticospinal fibers from the ipsilateral precentral gyrus and adjacent areas of cerebral cortex.

Important brainstem structures caudal to this level (i.e., between here and the spinal cord): pyramidal decussation (at the spinomedullary junction), where most fibers of the pyramids cross to form the lateral corticospinal tracts.

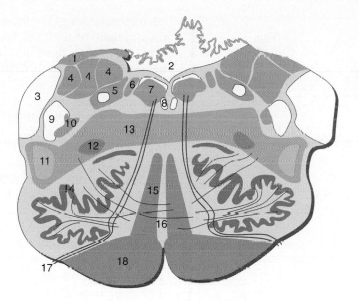

Figure 15-3   Rostral medulla.

Rostral Medulla

1. *Cochlear nuclei.* Second-order auditory neurons that project bilaterally to the superior olivary nucleus and into the lateral lemniscus.

2. *Fourth ventricle.* Continuous rostrally with the aqueduct and caudally with the central canal.

3. *Inferior cerebellar peduncle.* By the time it enters the cerebellum, it contains crossed olivocerebellar fibers, vestibulocerebellar fibers, most spinocerebellar fibers, and other cerebellar afferents.

4. *Vestibular nuclei.* Second-order neurons that form vestibulospinal tracts, much of the MLF, and projections to the cerebellum and thalamus.

5. *Nucleus of the solitary tract,* surrounding the solitary tract. This is much like a posterior column system for information from viscera and taste buds: Central branches of afferents from cranial nerves VII, IX, and X travel through the tract to reach the nucleus.

6. *Dorsal motor nucleus of the vagus.* Preganglionic parasympathetic neurons for thoracic and abdominal viscera.

7. *Hypoglossal nucleus.* Lower motor neurons for ipsilateral tongue muscles.

8. *Medial longitudinal fasciculus* (MLF). At this level, the fibers of the medial vestibulospinal tract.

9. *Spinal trigeminal tract.* Primary afferents from the ipsilateral side of the face, including those conveying information about pain and temperature to caudal parts of the spinal trigeminal nucleus.

10. *Spinal trigeminal nucleus.* Some neurons at intermediate levels like this are interneurons in the blink reflex arc.

11. *Anterolateral pathway.* Mostly crossed fibers of second-order spinal neurons conveying pain and temperature information to the thalamus (spinothalamic tract), reticular formation, and midbrain.

12. *Location of nucleus ambiguus.* Lower motor neurons for laryngeal and pharyngeal muscles (also contains preganglionic parasympathetic neurons for the heart).

13. *Reticular formation.*

14. *Inferior olivary nucleus.* Gives rise to climbing fibers that end in the contralateral half of the cerebellum (see Chapter 20).

15. *Medial lemniscus,* the principal ascending pathway for tactile and proprioceptive information. Originates in the contralateral posterior column nuclei and terminates in the thalamus (VPL).

16. *Raphe nuclei.* Serotonergic neurons that at this level are one source of descending pain-control fibers to the spinal cord.

17. *Hypoglossal nerve fibers,* on their way to ipsilateral tongue muscles.

18. *Pyramid.* Corticospinal fibers from the ipsilateral precentral gyrus and adjacent areas of cerebral cortex.

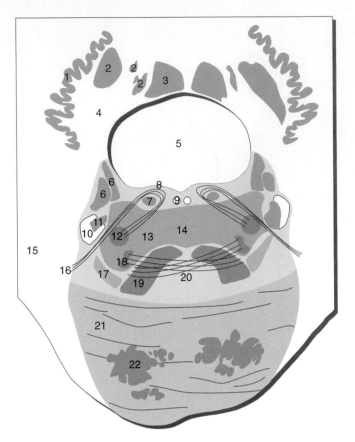

Figure 15-4   Caudal pons.

Caudal Pons

1. *Dentate nucleus.* The deep nucleus connected to the lateral part of the cerebellar hemisphere and the source of most of the fibers in the superior cerebellar peduncle (see Chapter 20).

2. *Interposed nucleus.* The deep cerebellar nucleus connected to the medial part of the cerebellar hemisphere and the source of most of the remaining fibers in the superior cerebellar peduncle (see Chapter 20).

3. *Fastigial nucleus.* The deep cerebellar nucleus connected to the cerebellar vermis (see Chapter 20).

4. *Superior cerebellar peduncle,* just forming in the cerebellum. The principal output pathway from the cerebellum.

5. *Fourth ventricle.* Continuous rostrally with the aqueduct and caudally with the central canal.

6. *Vestibular nuclei.* Second-order neurons that form vestibulospinal tracts, much of the MLF, and projections to the cerebellum and thalamus.

7. *Abducens nucleus.* Lower motor neurons for the ipsilateral lateral rectus, as well as the interneurons that project through the contralateral MLF to medial rectus motor neurons.

8. *Internal genu of the facial nerve.* Facial nerve fibers, most of them on their way to ipsilateral muscles of facial expression, that hook around the abducens nucleus before leaving the brainstem.

9. *Medial longitudinal fasciculus (MLF).* At this level, fibers from vestibular nuclei and abducens interneurons, active in coordinating eye movements.

10. *Spinal trigeminal tract.* Primary afferents from the ipsilateral side of the face, including those conveying information about pain and temperature to caudal parts of the spinal trigeminal nucleus.

11. *Spinal trigeminal nucleus.* Some primary afferents of the spinal trigeminal tract, particularly those carrying tactile information, end at this relatively rostral level.

12. *Facial motor nucleus.* Lower motor neurons for ipsilateral muscles of facial expression.

13. *Reticular formation.*

14. *Raphe nuclei.* Widely projecting serotonergic neurons that collectively blanket the CNS. Those in intermediate brainstem levels like this are one source of descending pain-control fibers to the spinal cord, and also project to other brainstem levels and the cerebellum.

15. *Middle cerebellar peduncle.* Fibers from contralateral pontine nuclei that end as mossy fibers (see Chapter 20) in all areas of cerebellar cortex.

16. *Facial nerve fibers.* Most of them are on their way to ipsilateral muscles of facial expression.

17. *Anterolateral pathway.* Mostly crossed fibers of second-order spinal neurons conveying pain and temperature information to the thalamus (spinothalamic tract), reticular formation, and midbrain. At this level, it also includes a contribution from the spinal trigeminal nucleus.

18. *Superior olivary nucleus.* First site of convergence of fibers representing the two ears and the source of many of the fibers of the lateral lemniscus.

19. *Medial lemniscus,* the principal ascending pathway for tactile and proprioceptive information. Originates in the contralateral posterior column nuclei and terminates in the thalamus (VPL).

20. *Trapezoid body.* Crossing auditory fibers, primarily from the cochlear nuclei.

21. *Pontine nuclei and pontocerebellar fibers.* Efferents from the cerebral cortex descend through the cerebral peduncle to reach ipsilateral pontine nuclei, whose axons cross in the basal pons and form the contralateral middle cerebellar peduncle.

22. *Corticospinal, corticobulbar, and corticopontine fibers,* from ipsilateral cerebral cortex.

Important brainstem structures between Figures 15-4 and 15-3, near the pontomedullary junction: cochlear nuclei (just beginning in Fig. 15-3), the second-order neurons of the auditory pathway; inferior cerebellar peduncle enters the cerebellum; attachment points of the abducens, facial, and vestibulocochlear nerves.

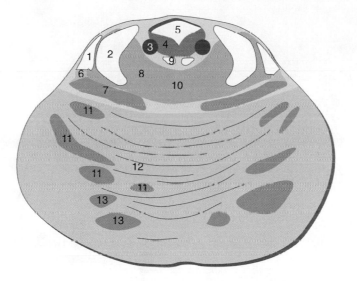

Figure 15-5 Rostral pons.

Rostral Pons

1. *Lateral lemniscus.* Ascending auditory fibers from the cochlear and superior olivary nuclei, representing both ears.

2. *Superior cerebellar peduncle.* The principal output pathway from the cerebellum.

3. *Locus ceruleus.* Widely projecting noradrenergic neurons that collectively blanket the CNS.

4. *Periventricular gray.* Continuous with the periaqueductal gray, the site of origin of the descending pain control pathway that relays in raphe nuclei of the rostral medulla and caudal pons (among other connections).

5. *Fourth ventricle* (rostral end, near the aqueduct).

6. *Anterolateral pathway.* Mostly crossed fibers of second-order spinal neurons conveying pain and temperature information to the thalamus (spinothalamic tract), reticular formation, and midbrain. At this level, it also includes a contribution from the spinal trigeminal nucleus.

7. *Medial lemniscus,* the principal ascending pathway for tactile and proprioceptive information. Originates in the contralateral posterior column nuclei and terminates in the thalamus (VPL). At this level, it also includes a contribution from the trigeminal main sensory nucleus on its way to VPM.

8. *Reticular formation.*

9. *Medial longitudinal fasciculus (MLF).* At this level, fibers from vestibular nuclei and abducens interneurons, active in coordinating eye movements.

10. *Raphe nuclei.* Widely projecting serotonergic neurons that collectively blanket the CNS. Those in rostral brainstem levels like this project mainly to the cerebrum and cerebellum.

11. *Corticopontine fibers,* from ipsilateral cerebral cortex.

12. *Pontine nuclei and pontocerebellar fibers.* Efferents from the cerebral cortex descend through the cerebral peduncle to reach ipsilateral pontine nuclei, whose axons cross in the basal pons and form the contralateral middle cerebellar peduncle.

13. *Corticospinal and corticobulbar fibers,* from the ipsilateral precentral gyrus and adjacent cortical areas.

Important brainstem structures between Figures 15-5 and 15-4: trigeminal main sensory nucleus (midpons), the second-order neurons for large-diameter trigeminal afferents; trigeminal motor nucleus (midpons), the lower motor neurons for muscles of mastication.

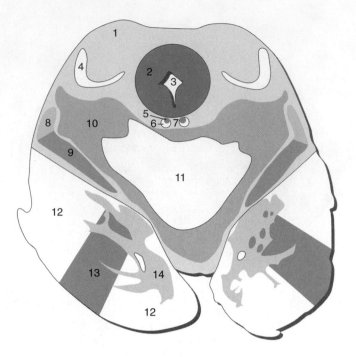

Figure 15-6   Caudal midbrain.

Caudal Midbrain

1. *Inferior colliculus*. A stop in the auditory pathway where the lateral lemniscus ends and the brachium of the inferior colliculus begins, in turn carrying auditory information to the medial geniculate nucleus of the thalamus.

2. *Periaqueductal gray*. Site of origin of the descending pain control pathway that relays in raphe nuclei of the rostral medulla and caudal pons (among other connections).

3. *Cerebral aqueduct*, continuous rostrally with the third ventricle and caudally with the fourth ventricle.

4. *Lateral lemniscus ending in the inferior colliculus*, the next stop in the central auditory pathway.

5. *Trochlear nucleus*. Lower motor neurons for the contralateral superior oblique muscle.

6. *Medial longitudinal fasciculus (MLF)*. At this level, fibers from vestibular nuclei and abducens interneurons, active in coordinating eye movements.

7. *Raphe nuclei*. Widely projecting serotonergic neurons that collectively blanket the CNS. Those in rostral brainstem levels like this project mainly to the cerebrum.

8. *Anterolateral pathway*. Mostly crossed fibers of second-order spinal neurons conveying pain and temperature information to the thalamus (spinothalamic tract), reticular formation, and midbrain. At this level, it also includes a contribution from the spinal trigeminal nucleus.

9. *Medial lemniscus*, the principal ascending pathway for tactile and proprioceptive information. Originates in the contralateral posterior column nuclei and terminates in the thalamus (VPL). At this level, it also includes a contribution from the trigeminal main sensory nucleus on its way to VPM.

10. *Reticular formation*.

11. *Decussation of the superior cerebellar peduncles*. Cerebellar output fibers crossing on their way to the red nucleus and thalamus (VL).

12. *Corticopontine fibers* from ipsilateral cerebral cortex, in the cerebral peduncle.

13. *Corticospinal and corticobulbar fibers* from the ipsilateral precentral gyrus and adjacent cortical areas.

14. Last few *pontine nuclei*. Source of pontocerebellar fibers that cross the midline and form the middle cerebellar peduncle.

Important brainstem structures between Figures 15-6 and 15-5: Trochlear nerves decussate and exit from the dorsal surface of the brainstem (pons-midbrain junction).

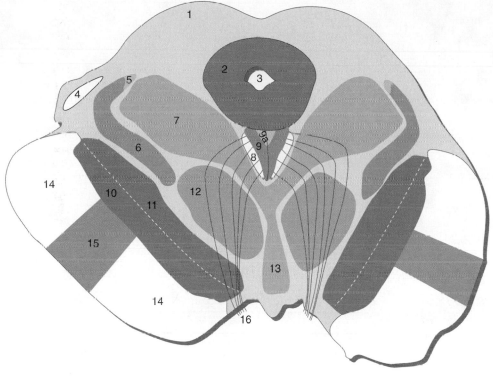

Figure 15-7 Rostral midbrain.

Rostral Midbrain

1. *Superior colliculus.* Involved in visual attention and eye movements. Inputs from the retina and visual cortex reach it through the brachium of the superior colliculus.

2. *Periaqueductal gray.* Site of origin of the descending pain control pathway that relays in raphe nuclei of the rostral medulla and caudal pons (among other connections).

3. *Cerebral aqueduct,* continuous rostrally with the third ventricle and caudally with the fourth ventricle.

4. *Brachium of the inferior colliculus.* Ascending auditory fibers on their way from the inferior colliculus to the medial geniculate nucleus of the thalamus.

5. *Anterolateral pathway.* Mostly crossed fibers of second-order spinal neurons conveying pain and temperature information to the thalamus (spinothalamic tract), reticular formation, and midbrain. At this level, it also includes a contribution from the spinal trigeminal nucleus.

6. *Medial lemniscus,* the principal ascending pathway for tactile and proprioceptive information. Originates in the contralateral posterior column nuclei and terminates in the thalamus (VPL). At this level, it also includes a contribution from the trigeminal main sensory nucleus on its way to VPM.

7. *Reticular formation.*

8. Last of the *medial longitudinal fasciculus (MLF),* conveying information from vestibular nuclei and abducens interneurons to the oculomotor nucleus.

9. *Oculomotor nucleus.* Lower motor neurons for most extraocular muscles.

9a. *Edinger-Westphal nucleus*; preganglionic parasympathetic component of the oculomotor nucleus, supplying the pupillary sphincter and the ciliary muscle.

10. *Substantia nigra* (reticular part). Inputs from the caudate nucleus and putamen, outputs to the thalamus and other sites (see Chapter 19).

11. *Substantia nigra* (compact part). Dopaminergic neurons whose axons terminate in the caudate nucleus and putamen.

12. *Red nucleus.* Interconnected with cerebellar circuitry, and the source of the small rubrospinal tract (see Chapter 20).

13. *Ventral tegmental area.* Dopaminergic neurons whose axons terminate in limbic and frontal cortical sites.

14. *Corticopontine fibers* from ipsilateral cerebral cortex, in the cerebral peduncle.

15. *Corticospinal and corticobulbar fibers* from the ipsilateral precentral gyrus and adjacent cortical areas.

16. *Oculomotor nerve fibers.*

The Thalamus and Internal Capsule: Getting to and from the Cerebral Cortex

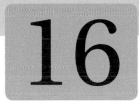

The **diencephalon** is a relatively small, centrally located part of the cerebrum that, like the spinal cord and brainstem, is functionally important way out of proportion to its size. It is subdivided into four general regions, each with the term "thalamus" as all or part of its name.

The Diencephalon Includes the Epithalamus, Subthalamus, Hypothalamus, and Thalamus

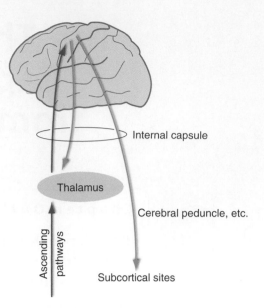

Figure 16-1 Overview of cortical connections with subcortical sites.

Key Concepts

The epithalamus includes the pineal gland.
The subthalamus includes the subthalamic nucleus.

The major components of the diencephalon, the **thalamus** and **hypothalamus**, are active in practically everything we do. The thalamus is the gateway to the cerebral cortex and the principal subject of this chapter. The hypothalamus regulates autonomic functions and drive-related behavior and is discussed further in Chapter 23.

The **epithalamus** and **subthalamus** are located where their names imply—above and below the thalamus, respectively. The major constituent of the epithalamus is the **pineal gland**, an endocrine gland near the posterior commissure and the midbrain-diencephalon junction. It secretes melatonin, a hormone involved in the regulation of circadian rhythms and seasonal cycles. The major constituent of the subthalamus is the **subthalamic nucleus**, an important part of the basal ganglia (Chapter 19).

The Thalamus Is the Gateway to the Cerebral Cortex

Some collections of chemically coded fibers, such as serotonergic fibers from the raphe nuclei and noradrenergic fibers from the locus ceruleus, reach the cerebral cortex directly. However, the vast majority of the afferents to the cerebral cortex arise either in the cortex itself or in the thalamus. **Thalamocortical** afferents include fibers representing all the specific sensory, motor, and limbic pathways. In contrast, efferents from the cerebral cortex to sites like the spinal cord, brainstem, and basal ganglia reach their targets directly. (Although there are also many cortical projections back to the thalamus, these do not form a link in any descending pathway.) This large collection of thalamocortical afferents and cortical efferents travels through the **internal capsule** (Fig. 16-1).

The Thalamus Has Anterior, Medial, and Lateral Divisions, Defined by the Internal Medullary Lamina

A thin sheet of myelinated fibers, the **internal medullary lamina**, subdivides the thalamus into nuclear groups. The internal medullary lamina bifurcates anteriorly and so defines **anterior**, **medial**, and **lateral** nuclear groups (Fig. 16-2).

The anterior and medial subdivisions have only one major nucleus each (the **anterior** and **dorsomedial** nuclei, respectively). The lateral division, in contrast, contains an array of four major nuclei or nuclear groups. From anterior to posterior these are the **ventral anterior** nucleus (**VA**), the **ventral lateral** nucleus (**VL**), the **ventral posterolateral** and **ventral posteromedial** nuclei (**VPL** and **VPM**), and the **pulvinar** (Fig. 16-3). In addition, the **lateral** and **medial geniculate** nuclei (**LGN** and **MGN**) form two bumps posteriorly and inferiorly on the main bulk of the thalamus.

midline

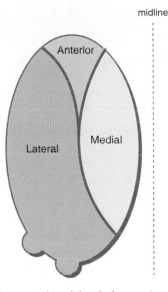

Figure 16-2   Topography of the thalamus, in a schematic axial section.

Intralaminar Nuclei Are Embedded in the Internal Medullary Lamina

Clumps of cells embedded in the internal medullary lamina collectively constitute the **intralaminar nuclei**, which have a distinctive pattern of connections (THB6

midline

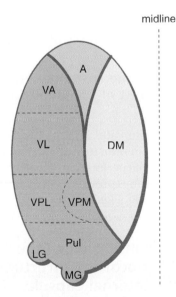

Figure 16-3   Principal thalamic nuclei. This schematic axial section was drawn as though most of the thalamus had been squashed into this one plane. For example, the anterior nucleus is toward the top of the thalamus and the geniculates are toward the bottom; all are not actually present in the same axial plane. *A,* Anterior nucleus; *DM,* dorsomedial nucleus; *LG,* lateral geniculate nucleus; *MG,* medial geniculate nucleus; *Pul,* pulvinar; *VA,* ventral anterior nucleus; *VL,* ventral lateral nucleus; *VPL,* ventral posterolateral nucleus; *VPM,* ventral posteromedial nucleus.

Figure 16-14D, p. 402). Functionally similar collections of neurons on the ventricular surface of the thalamus are called the **midline nuclei**.

The Thalamic Reticular Nucleus Partially Surrounds the Thalamus

A thin shell of neurons, called the **reticular nucleus**, covers the lateral and anterior surfaces of the thalamus. The reticular nucleus is spoken of as part of the thalamus because of its location, but in terms of development and connections (THB6 Figure 16-19, p. 406) it is actually a separate structure. (It shares the name "reticular" with the reticular formation of the brainstem because of its reticulated appearance, but these two are actually distinct entities.)

Patterns of Input and Output Connections Define Functional Categories of Thalamic Nuclei

> **Key Concept**
>
> All thalamic nuclei (except the reticular nucleus) are variations on a common theme.

If the thalamus were just a simple relay through which information reached the cerebral cortex, there would be little point in having one. In fact, its major function is as a gateway where determinations are made about which information should reach the cortex. This is accomplished by a common wiring scheme for all thalamic nuclei (except the reticular nucleus), involving two sets of inputs: **regulatory inputs** that determine the functional state of thalamic neurons and **specific inputs** that specify the kind of information a given thalamic neuron can pass on to the cortex when appropriate. The regulatory inputs are broadly similar for all thalamic nuclei (except the reticular nucleus), arising in the brainstem reticular formation, the thalamic reticular nucleus, and the cerebral cortex itself.

Thalamic nuclei that receive most of their specific inputs from subcortical structures are **relay nuclei** (Fig. 16-4); the medial geniculate nucleus, for example, receives most of its specific inputs from the inferior colliculus and relays this information to auditory cortex. (The intralaminar and midline nuclei also receive specific inputs from subcortical sites, in this case parts of the basal ganglia and limbic system, but send more outputs to the basal ganglia and limbic system than to cerebral cortex; their functional role is not well understood.) Thalamic nuclei that receive most of their specific inputs from the cerebral cortex are **association nuclei**, which are important for distributing information between different cortical areas (Fig. 16-5).

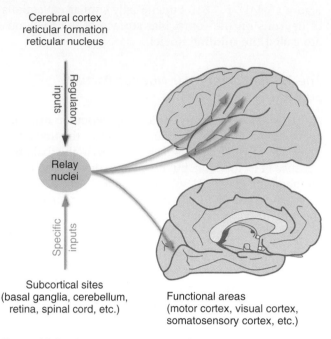

Figure 16-4 Connection patterns of thalamic relay nuclei.

Thalamic Projection Neurons Have Two Physiological States

The regulatory inputs to thalamic neurons are able to switch them back and forth between two states, one in which these neurons are able to transmit information accurately to their cortical targets and one in which instead they fire periodic bursts of action potentials (THB6 Figure 16-15, p. 403). Thalamic neurons are in this **bursting** state during some phases of sleep and probably during periods of inattention. A major mechanism of focusing attention is thought to be using regulatory inputs to switch thalamic neurons from the bursting mode into the accurate-transmission (**tonic**) mode.

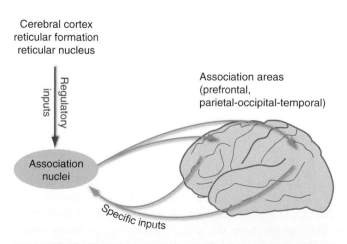

Figure 16-5 Connection patterns of thalamic association nuclei.

There Are Relay Nuclei for Sensory, Motor, and Limbic Systems

Thalamic relay nuclei are part of specific functional systems, receiving particular bundles of afferents and projecting heavily to particular cortical areas with more or less well-defined functions. The major examples of specific relay nuclei, with their inputs and outputs, are indicated in Fig. 16-6.

The Dorsomedial Nucleus and Pulvinar Are the Principal Association Nuclei

Most of the cortical areas not accounted for in the projections of the thalamic relay nuclei form two large expanses of **association cortex** (see Chapter 22). The first, **prefrontal** association cortex, is located anterior to the motor areas of the frontal lobe. The second is the **parietal-occipital-temporal** association cortex. Each of these fields of association cortex receives major inputs from its own thalamic association nucleus, prefrontal areas from the dorsomedial nucleus and more posterior areas from the pulvinar.

The Thalamic Reticular Nucleus Projects to Other Thalamic Nuclei and Not to the Cerebral Cortex

The thalamic reticular nucleus is different from all other thalamic nuclei in that, rather than being a source of thalamocortical fibers, its GABAergic neurons are a major source of regulatory inputs to the rest of the thalamus.

Small Branches of the Posterior Cerebral Artery Provide Most of the Blood Supply to the Thalamus

The basilar artery bifurcates into the two posterior cerebral arteries directly inferior to the thalamus (THB6 Figure 6-10, p. 130), and small perforating or ganglionic branches of the posterior cerebrals provide most of the blood supply to the thalamus (THB6 Figure 16-20, p. 406).

Interconnections between the Cerebral Cortex and Subcortical Structures Travel through the Internal Capsule

Key Concepts

The internal capsule has five parts.

Most cortical afferents and efferents travel through the internal capsule, a bundle of fibers compacted between the lenticular nucleus (lateral to it) and the thalamus

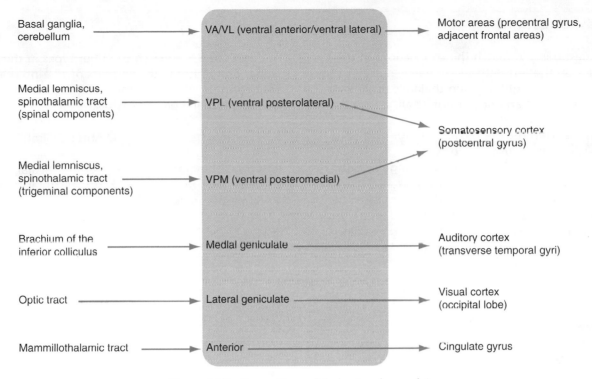

Figure 16-6 Connections of thalamic relay nuclei.

and head of the caudate (medial to it). (Its three-dimensional shape can be seen in THB6 Figure 16-23, p. 410.)

Different parts of the internal capsule are named for their relationship with the lenticular nucleus. The **anterior limb** travels between the lenticular nucleus and the head of the caudate and the **posterior limb** between the lenticular nucleus and the thalamus; the **genu** is the region at the junction of the anterior and posterior limbs. The internal capsule actually wraps partly around the lenticular nucleus; the **retrolenticular part** is just behind it, and the **sublenticular part** dips under the most posterior part of the lenticular nucleus.

The major contents of the various parts of the internal capsule can be inferred, for the most part, from their positions relative to various thalamic nuclei and cortical areas (Table 16-1; see THB6 Figures 16-24 and 16-25, pp. 411 and 412).

Small Branches of the Middle Cerebral Artery Provide Most of the Blood Supply to the Internal Capsule

The internal capsule is lateral to the thalamus and extends anterior to it. Corresponding to this anatomical location, the blood supply to the internal capsule is mostly from small perforating or ganglionic branches of the middle and anterior cerebral arteries (THB6 Figure 16-20, p. 406).

Table 16-1	Contents of the internal capsule*		
Portion	**Origin**	**Termination**	**Other Names**
Anterior limb	Anterior nucleus	Cingulate gyrus	
	Dorsomedial nucleus	Prefrontal cortex	
Posterior limb	Motor cortex	Spinal cord	Corticospinal tract
	Motor cortex	Brainstem	Corticobulbar, corticopontine[†] tracts
	VPL/VPM	Postcentral gyrus	Somatosensory radiation
Retrolenticular part	Pulvinar	Association cortex	
	LGN	Visual cortex	Optic radiation
Sublenticular part	Pulvinar	Association cortex	
	LGN	Visual cortex	Optic radiation
	MGN	Auditory cortex	Auditory radiation

*The genu is not included because it is a transition zone between the anterior and posterior limbs and has no distinctive contents of its own.
[†]Actually comes from more than just motor cortex; see Chapter 20.

Study Questions

For questions 1-7, match the connections in the column on the left with the thalamic nuclei in the column on the right; a given thalamic nucleus may be used more than once or not at all.

1. Inputs from the medial lemniscus
2. Outputs to prefrontal cortex
3. Outputs to the occipital lobe
4. Outputs to the postcentral gyrus
5. Inputs from the mammillothalamic tract
6. Outputs to the transverse temporal gyri
7. Outputs to the precentral gyrus

a. Anterior nucleus
b. VL
c. Medial geniculate nucleus
d. Dorsomedial nucleus
e. VPL
f. Lateral geniculate nucleus

For questions 8-11, match the fiber types in the column on the left with the parts of the internal capsule in the column on the right; for each fiber type, use as many parts as apply.

8. Efferents from the anterior nucleus
9. Corticospinal tract
10. Optic radiation
11. Somatosensory fibers

a. Anterior limb
b. Posterior limb
c. Retrolenticular part
d. Sublenticular part

The Visual System

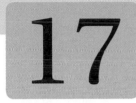

The visual system is the most studied sensory system, partly because we are such a visually oriented species and partly because of its relative simplicity. In addition, the visual pathway is highly organized in a topographical sense, so even though it stretches from the front of your face to the back of your head, damage anyplace causes deficits that are relatively easy to understand.

The Eye Has Three Concentric Tissue Layers and a Lens

Vertebrate eyes perform functions analogous to those performed by cameras, but do so using three roughly spherical, concentric tissue layers either derived from or comparable to the dura mater, the pia-arachnoid, and the CNS (Fig. 17-1). The thick, collagenous outer layer forms the **sclera**—the white of the eye—and continues anteriorly as the **cornea** and posteriorly as the dural **optic nerve sheath**. The middle layer is loose, vascular connective tissue that forms the pigmented **choroid** that lines the sclera; it continues anteriorly as the vascular core of the **ciliary body**, the **ciliary muscle**, and most of the **iris**. The innermost layer, itself a double layer because of the way the eye develops (THB6 Figure 17-1, p. 416), forms the **neural retina** (closer to the interior of the eye) and the **retinal pigment epithelium** (adjacent to the choroid); it continues anteriorly as the double-layered epithelial covering of the ciliary body and the posterior surface of the iris. Suspended inside the eye, and not really part of any of these tissue layers, is the **lens**.

Collectively, structures derived from these three layers, together with the lens, take care of the functions dealt with by cameras: keeping a photosensitive surface in a stable position, focusing images of objects at different distances onto this surface, regulating the amount of light that reaches the photosensitive surface, and absorbing stray light.

Intraocular Pressure Maintains the Shape of the Eye

The shape of the eye is maintained by having it blown up like a soccer ball. The sclera and cornea provide the tough wall, and the inflation pressure is generated by a fluid secretion-reabsorption system much like the CSF system. The **ciliary epithelium** secretes a CSF-like **aqueous humor** into the **posterior chamber** (the space between the iris and the lens). Just as CSF circulates through the ventricles and subarachnoid space and then filters through arachnoid villi, aqueous humor moves through the **pupil**, into the **anterior chamber** (between the iris and cornea), gets filtered into a **scleral venous sinus** (the **canal of Schlemm**) near the corneoscleral junction, and from there reaches the venous system. The resistance to flow at the filtration site results in a pressure buildup in the aqueous humor. Because the space behind the lens is filled with gelatinous, incompressible **vitreous humor**, the pressure in the aqueous humor is transmitted throughout the interior of the eye and the shape of the eye is maintained.

The Cornea and Lens Focus Images on the Retina

There's a big change in refractive index at the interface between air and the front of the cornea, so this is where most of the focusing happens. The lens contributes less because there's much less change in refractive index going from aqueous humor to lens or from lens to vitreous humor. The major importance of the lens is in adjusting the focus of the eye during **accommodation**

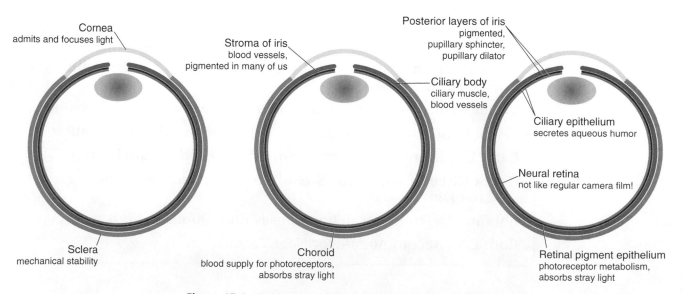

Figure 17-1 Derivatives of the three tissue layers of the eye.

for near vision (see Fig. 17-9 later in this chapter). Contraction of the ciliary muscle relaxes some of the tension on the capsule suspending the lens, allowing the lens to get fatter and the eye to focus on near objects.

The Iris Affects the Brightness and Quality of the Image Focused on the Retina

The pigmented posterior epithelial layers of the iris prevent light from getting into the eye except through the pupil, so regulating the size of the pupil regulates the amount of light reaching the retina (although neural changes in the retina are much more important for regulating the sensitivity of the eye). The **pupillary sphincter**, innervated by the oculomotor nerve via the ciliary ganglion, makes the pupil smaller (see Figs. 17-7 and 17-8 later in this chapter). The **pupillary dilator**, innervated by upper thoracic sympathetics via the superior cervical ganglion, makes the pupil larger.

A System of Barriers Partially Separates the Retina from the Rest of the Body

Another indication that the neural retina is really an outgrowth of the CNS is the way its neurons are protected by a similar three-part barrier system. The endothelial cells of retinal capillaries are zipped up by tight junctions, forming a **blood-retinal barrier** system in the literal sense. The ciliary epithelium, just like the choroid epithelium, prevents diffusion from the ciliary body into aqueous humor. Finally, the retinal pigment epithelium, in a way analogous to the barrier function of the arachnoid, prevents diffusion from the choroid into the retina.

The Retina Contains Five Major Neuronal Cell Types

> ### Key Concept
>
> Retinal neurons and synapses are arranged in layers.

The job of the retina is to convert patterns of light into trains of action potentials in the **optic nerve**. It does this using five basic cell types (Fig. 17-2), whose cell bodies are arranged in three layers (**outer** and **inner nuclear layers**, **ganglion cell layer**). Alternating with these three layers of cell bodies are an **outer** and an **inner plexiform layer** where the synaptic interactions occur. In the outer plexiform layer, photoreceptor cells (**rods** and **cones**) bring visual information in, **bipolar cells** take it out, and **horizontal cells** mediate lateral interactions. In the inner plexiform layer bipolar cells bring visual information in, ganglion cells take it out (their axons form the optic nerve), and **amacrine cells** mediate lateral interactions.

Standard descriptions of the retina as a 10-layered structure also include a row of junctions between adjacent photoreceptors (**outer limiting membrane**), the layer of ganglion cell axons (**nerve fiber layer**), and the basal lamina on the vitreal surface of the retina (**inner limiting membrane**). Oddly enough, the layers are

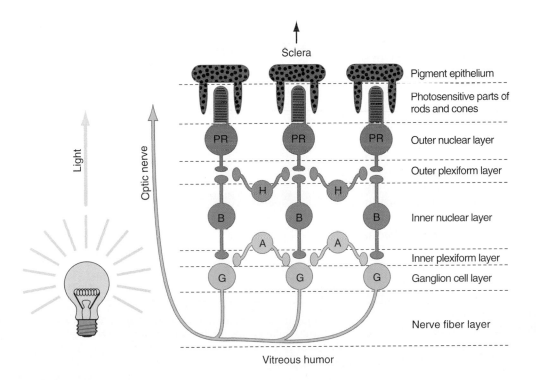

Figure 17-2 Organization of the retina. *A*, Amacrine cells; *B*, bipolar cells; *G*, ganglion cells; *H*, horizontal cells; *PR*, photoreceptor cells.

arranged so that the last part of vertebrate neural retinas reached by light is the photosensitive parts of the rod and cone cells, embedded in processes of pigment epithelial cells.

The Retina Is Regionally Specialized

Key Concepts

Rods function in dim light.
Populations of cones signal spatial detail and color.

Ganglion cell axons travel along the vitreal surface of the retina, and so they need to pierce the sclera to leave the eye in the optic nerve. They do so by converging on the **optic disk**, slightly medial to the optic axis, turning 90° posteriorly, and leaving the eye. Here the optic nerve acquires a dural (scleral) sheath continuous with the dural covering of the CNS. (The dural sheath is lined with arachnoid and contains a bit of subarachnoid space; increases in intracranial pressure are therefore transmitted along the optic nerve and cause **papilledema**, or swelling of the optic disk.) Because there are no photoreceptors at the optic disk, it corresponds to a **blind spot** in the visual field of each eye. The optics of the eye reverse images on the retina, so the blind spot of each eye lies near the horizontal meridian of the visual field, slightly *lateral* to the center of the field.

The center of the visual field corresponds to the **fovea**, a small retinal region in the middle of a pigmented zone called the **macula**. The fovea is filled with thin, densely packed cones and no rods. All the other neuronal types are pushed toward the periphery, so the center of the fovea is a small pit (THB6 Figure 17-11, p. 425). Outside the fovea, the number of cones diminishes quickly. The packing density of rods, in contrast, first increases rapidly and then declines slowly. We have three different types of cones in terms of the wavelength to which each is most sensitive, so the total cone population can be used for color vision. Rods, on the other hand, come in only one variety but function at lower light levels than do cones. The fovea, with its densely packed cones, is therefore specialized for high **spatial acuity** and **color vision**, but only at moderate or high levels of illumination. The region around the fovea, with many rods and few cones, has reasonably good spatial acuity, works at low light levels, but is not very useful for color vision. Finally, the peripheral retina, with few rods and even fewer cones, is mostly good for telling us that something is moving around out there.

Retinal Neurons Translate Patterns of Light into Patterns of Contrast

The retina, like camera film or the sensor in a digital camera, is photosensitive, but that's about as far as the similarity goes. Visual systems are designed to make things look the same to us whether they're up close or far away, dimly lit or brightly lit, at sunrise or midday. This is accomplished by a process that begins in the retina: Single optic nerve fibers report not so much on the actual illumination at some location in the visual field as on differences between the illumination at one location and neighboring locations. The result is that something like the edge of a letter looks pretty much the same whether we look at it in room light or sunlight.

Photopigments Are G Protein–Coupled Receptors That Cause Hyperpolarizing Receptor Potentials

Phototransduction is a lot like G protein–coupled synaptic transmission (Fig. 17-3); the equivalent of the postsynaptic receptor protein is **opsin**, which in the dark binds a particular stereoisomer of a vitamin A

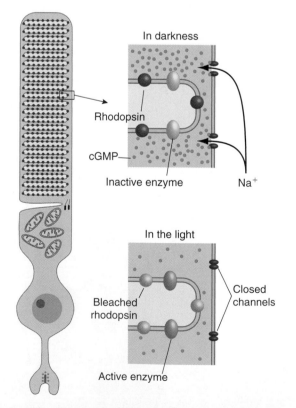

Figure 17-3 Phototransduction in rods. Even though the photopigment-studded membranous disks in cones are open to extracellular space, the transduction process is basically the same (see THB6 Figure 17-16B, p. 431).

derivative (**11-*cis*-retinal**). Absorption of a photon by a visual pigment molecule has only one direct effect: It **photoisomerizes** the 11-*cis*-retinal, changing the way it fits with opsin. This in turn activates nearby G proteins, each of which activates an enzyme that hydrolyzes cytoplasmic **cyclic guanosine monophosphate** (**cGMP**). The surface membranes of photoreceptor outer segments contain cGMP gated cation channels, so cGMP hydrolysis causes the channels to close and the photoreceptor to hyperpolarize. Hence, light for a photoreceptor is a lot like neurotransmitter release at an unusual G protein–coupled inhibitory synapse— in the light G proteins dissociate, the concentration of a second messenger changes, and cation channels close.

Ganglion Cells Have Center-Surround Receptive Fields

> ### Key Concept
> Center-surround receptive fields are formed in the outer plexiform layer.

Ganglion cells, as mentioned previously, are contrast detectors. The receptive field of each has a **center** and a **surround**. The center is a central spot where light causes the cell to fire faster (**ON-center**) or slower (**OFF-center**), and the surround is an area where light has just the opposite effect. The result is that if uniform illumination (the level doesn't matter) covers the whole receptive field, the center and surround more or less cancel each other out. In contrast, if the illumination is non-uniform, either the center or the surround will "win" and the ganglion cell will signal the difference between the two.

The centers of ganglion cell receptive fields result from "straight-through" transmission from receptors to bipolar cells to ganglion cells (Fig. 17-4). The surrounds result from lateral interactions mediated by horizontal and amacrine cells (especially horizontal cells).

Rod and Cone Signals Reach the Same Ganglion Cells

Even though we have one population of photoreceptors (rods) active in dim light and another population (cones) active in brighter light, it all gets signaled by a single population of ganglion cells. The exact way in which rod information reaches ganglion cells depends on the level of illumination; elaborate changes in some retinal synapses are regulated by light levels (THB6 Figure 17-25, p. 439).

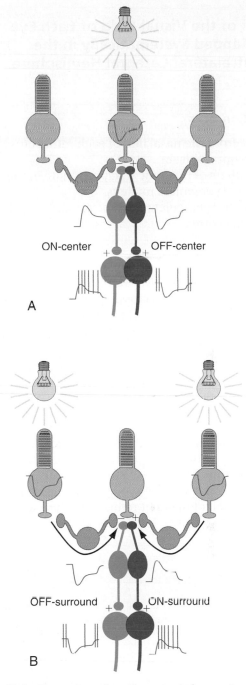

Figure 17-4 Formation of center-surround receptive fields in the outer plexiform layer. **A,** The centers are formed by transmission from photoreceptors to bipolar cells. Photoreceptors release less glutamate when illuminated. ON-center bipolar cells have inhibitory glutamate receptors (–), so the glutamate decrease causes them to depolarize. OFF-center bipolar cells have more typical excitatory glutamate receptors (+), so the glutamate decrease causes them to hyperpolarize. Bipolar to ganglion cell transmission is all excitatory (+). **B,** Illumination of photoreceptors also sends a signal through horizontal cells, causing neighboring photoreceptors to release *more* glutamate. This is the basis of the surround effect, producing an effect exactly the opposite of light in the center of the receptive field.

Half of the Visual Field of Each Eye Is Mapped Systematically in the Contralateral Cerebral Hemisphere

Key Concepts

Fibers from the nasal half of each retina cross in the optic chiasm.

Most fibers of the optic tract terminate in the lateral geniculate nucleus.

The lateral geniculate nucleus projects to primary visual cortex.

The central visual pathway has two important anatomical tasks, one related to crossings of the midline and the other to maps.

Because our eyes face forward their **visual fields** overlap to a great extent (THB6 Figure 17-32, p. 445), so it would make sense for information from each retina about the contralateral half of the visual world to reach a given side of the brain. This is neatly taken care of by a partial decussation of the optic nerves in the **optic chiasm**, in which the ganglion cell axons from the nasal half of each retina cross the midline and join undecussated fibers from the temporal half of the other retina in the **optic tract**. (For example, because the optics of the eye reverse things, the temporal half of the left retina and the nasal half of the right retina both "look at" the right

half of the visual world.) This separation of the visual world into two halves is maintained in the rest of the visual pathway. The optic tract ends in the **lateral geniculate nucleus** of the thalamus. The lateral geniculate gives rise to the **optic radiation**, which passes through the retrolenticular and sublenticular parts of the internal capsule and ends in **primary visual cortex** above and below the calcarine sulcus.

As in the case of other sensory systems, the visual system maintains an orderly map of the information it carries and emphasizes in this map certain functionally important regions. In this case, the visual pathway maintains a **retinotopic** map of the image falling on each retina, with a disproportionately large number of fibers representing the fovea. The mapping culminates in primary visual cortex, where the *retina* is represented right side up (i.e., superior *fields* below the calcarine sulcus, inferior fields above), the fovea posteriorly at the occipital pole and the periphery anteriorly (THB6 Figure 17-29, p. 443). The foveal representation, relative to the size of the fovea, is much larger than the representation of the periphery.

Damage at Different Points in the Visual Pathway Results in Predictable Deficits

Knowledge of the visual pathway enables you to predict the deficits resulting from damage anyplace in the pathway; knowledge of a little terminology allows you to name them (Fig. 17-5) and bewilder the uninitiated. Deficits are generally named for the visual field affected. **Heteronymous** means the affected fields of the two eyes

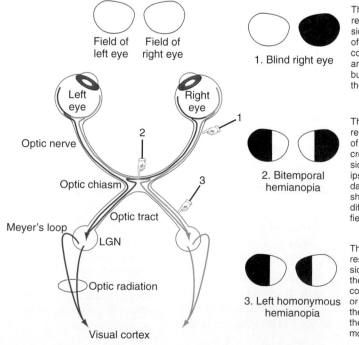

Field of left eye   Field of right eye

Left eye   Right eye

Optic nerve

Optic chiasm

Meyer's loop

Optic tract

LGN

Optic radiation

Visual cortex

1

2

3

1. Blind right eye

The maximum deficit that could result from damage on the right side of the visual pathway in front of the optic chiasm. Partial damage could cause loss of sectors, loss of an area straddling the midline, etc., but could only involve the field of the right eye.

2. Bitemporal hemianopia

The maximum deficit that could result from damage in the middle of the optic chiasm, affecting the crossing fibers. Damage on one side of the chiasm could cause an ipsilateral nasal field loss, but damage anywhere in the chiasm should generally cause losses in different parts of the two eyes' fields.

3. Left homonymous hemianopia

The maximum deficit that could result from damage on the right side of the visual pathway behind the optic chiasm. Partial damage could cause loss of only quadrants or sectors, or spare the left half of the foveal field, but the losses in the two eyes' visual fields should more or less overlap.

Figure 17-5 Visual field deficits.

do not overlap and **homonymous** means the affected fields overlap to a greater or lesser degree. Therefore, damage in front of the optic chiasm affects only the eye ipsilateral to the damage, damage to the optic chiasm typically causes heteronymous deficits, and damage behind the chiasm causes homonymous deficits. Terms like **hemianopia** and **quadrantanopia** mean half or a quarter of a visual field is nonfunctional.

Fibers on their way to the upper bank of the calcarine sulcus go through the retrolenticular part of the internal capsule and straight back to the occipital lobe. Fibers on their way to the lower bank go through the sublenticular part and loop out into the temporal lobe (**Meyer's loop**) before turning posteriorly toward the occipital lobe (THB6 Figure 17-28, p. 442). Damage in the optic radiation or the occipital lobe sometimes spares part of the large foveal representation, resulting in **foveal** or **macular sparing**.

Some Fibers of the Optic Tract Terminate in the Superior Colliculus, Accessory Optic Nuclei, and Hypothalamus

Although most ganglion cell axons terminate in the lateral geniculate nucleus, a smaller number reach other sites: the **superior colliculus** (orientation to visual stimuli), the nearby **pretectal area** (pupillary light reflex), other nearby **accessory optic nuclei** (reflex eye movements), and the **suprachiasmatic nucleus** of the hypothalamus (entraining circadian rhythms).

Primary Visual Cortex Sorts Visual Information and Distributes It to Other Cortical Areas

An important strategy used by the brain in information processing is to pick something apart into subcomponents and work on these separately. In visual processing this means dissecting the patterns of illumination coming from different parts of the visual field into their component elements—color, movement, borders, etc. This process begins way back in the retina, where small (and numerous) ganglion cells are particularly sensitive to colors and edges but other, larger ganglion cells are more sensitive to movement.

Visual Cortex Has a Columnar Organization

A major function of visual cortex is to continue this process of sorting out the different elements of a visual stimulus. Visual cortex is made up of a series of modules, each made up of a number of **columns** of neurons extending through the cortex. Collectively the columns of a module receive all the visual information from some

area of the contralateral visual field—a large area for modules in the peripheral part of the retinotopic map and a small area for modules in the foveal part (THB6 Figure 17-35, p. 449). The neurons in a given column have similar properties: they all respond best to stimuli in a particular part of the visual field, usually are more sensitive to input from one eye or the other, and typically have some other preference in common as well (color, movement in some direction, orientation of a border, etc.).

Visual Information Is Distributed in Dorsal and Ventral Streams

A second major function of visual cortex, once the various elements of visual stimuli have been sorted out, is to export information about these elements to specific areas of visual association cortex that are specialized to deal with them. Thus, there are visual association areas particularly interested in the color of an object, its distance from the eyes, details of its shape, the direction and velocity of movement, and other properties. Although the segregation of functions is far from complete, in general more dorsal areas process information about location and movement and more ventral areas process information about color and form (Fig. 17-6). As a result, rare, selective lesions in visual association areas can cause a selective loss of only some visual capabilities—even something as specific as the ability to recognize faces (THB6 Box 17-2, p. 451).

Early Experience Has Permanent Effects on the Visual System

The basic wiring pattern of the visual system is genetically determined and present at birth. However, there is a period of plasticity early in life during which visual experience is critical for refining and even maintaining these connections (see Chapter 24). Anything that interferes with normal binocular vision during this period (e.g., cataracts, misalignment of the eyes) can cause permanent changes in connections and permanent visual deficits. The duration of the **critical period** of plasticity varies from cortical area to area and from species to species, but may be as long as several years in humans.

Reflex Circuits Adjust the Size of the Pupil and the Focal Length of the Lens

The eye has its own equivalent of autoexposure and autofocus systems, based on muscles and reflex connections rather than photodiodes and motors.

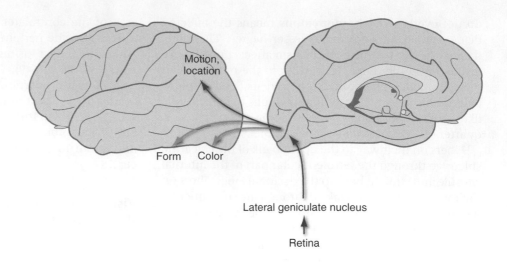

Figure 17-6   Dorsal and ventral streams in visual association cortex.

Illumination of Either Retina Causes Both Pupils to Constrict

The size of the pupil is determined by the balance between a relatively strong sphincter and a relatively weak dilator (Fig. 17-7). The sphincter receives parasympathetic innervation via the oculomotor nerve and the ciliary ganglion and is normally activated during the **pupillary light reflex** and the **near reflex** (next section). The dilator receives sympathetic innervation via the intermediolateral cell column of the spinal cord and the superior cervical ganglion. The preganglionic sympathetic neurons for the dilator can be activated by long descending pathways from the ipsilateral half of the hypothalamus, as well as by other routes.

Pupils of significantly unequal size usually signify damage to some aspect of the autonomic innervation of one eye or to the iris itself. A dilated pupil (**mydriasis**), unresponsive to all stimuli, could be caused by damage to the ipsilateral oculomotor nerve. Such damage, if it affected the entire nerve, would also be accompanied by weakness of the other muscles supplied by the third nerve, most prominently resulting in **ptosis** (because of a weak levator palpebrae) and lateral **strabismus** (because of an unopposed lateral rectus). A pupil that was relatively constricted (**miosis**), but still responsive to light shone through it, could be caused by damage to either its preganglionic or its postganglionic sympathetic innervation, or to fibers on the ipsilateral side of the brainstem as they descend from the hypothalamus to the spinal cord. (In the pons and medulla, the latter fibers are located near the spinothalamic tract.) This would constitute part of **Horner's syndrome** and would be accompanied by slight ipsilateral ptosis (weakness of the sympathetically innervated tarsal muscles) but not by any weakness of other extraocular muscles.

A commonly tested cranial nerve reflex is the pupillary light reflex (Fig. 17-8). Light shone through one pupil causes both sphincters to contract equally. The response of the illuminated eye is the **direct** reflex, and the equal response of the unilluminated eye is the **consensual**

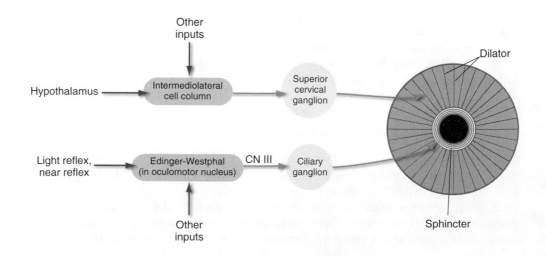

Figure 17-7   Control of pupil size.

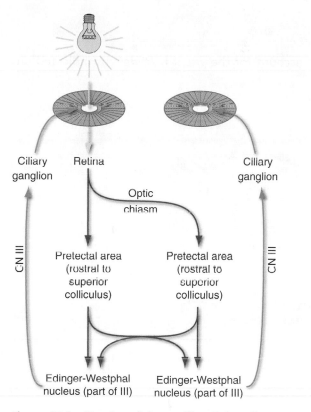

Figure 17-8   Circuitry of the pupillary light reflex.

Both Eyes Accommodate for Near Vision

Looking at something nearby causes three things to happen in reflex fashion: (1) Both medial recti contract, **converging** the eyes; (2) both ciliary muscles contract, allowing the lens to fatten (**accommodation**) and thus focus the image of the nearby object on the two retinas; and (3) both pupillary sphincters contract, improving the optical performance of the eye. Because this near reflex or accommodation reflex typically involves consciously looking at something, it is not surprising that its pathway involves a loop through visual cortex (Fig. 17-9). The afferent limb is the standard visual pathway through the lateral geniculate nucleus and visual cortex. After one or more synapses in the occipital lobe, the efferent limb involves a projection back through the brachium of the superior colliculus to the pretectal area and/or the superior colliculus and from there to the oculomotor nucleus. (The stop in the superior colliculus is omitted from Fig. 17-9 for simplicity.)

reflex. Afferent impulses for this reflex arc travel along ganglion cell axons in the optic nerve; half of these cross in the optic chiasm. However, they bypass the lateral geniculate nucleus and travel instead through the **brachium of the superior colliculus** to the **pretectal area**, just rostral to the superior colliculus at the midbrain-diencephalon junction. Fibers from the pretectal area then distribute bilaterally to the **Edinger-Westphal** subnucleus of the oculomotor nucleus, where the preganglionic parasympathetic neurons live. Because of the bilateral distribution of fibers both in the optic chiasm and in going from each pretectal area to the oculomotor nuclei, light in one eye causes equal constriction of both pupils. Optic nerve damage produces equal pupils, neither one of which responds to light shone into the eye ipsilateral to the damage, but both of which respond normally to light shone into the contralateral eye. Oculomotor nerve damage, in contrast, causes a dilated ipsilateral pupil that does not respond to light shone into either eye.

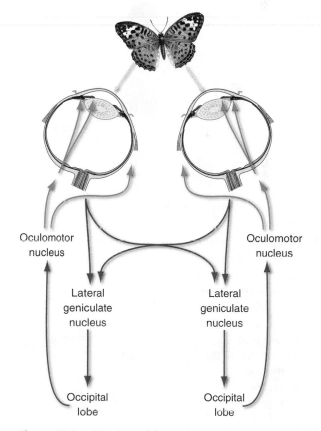

Figure 17-9   Circuitry of the accommodation (near) reflex.

Study Questions

For questions 1-6 choose the lesion site (*A-M*) most likely to account for the visual field deficits indicated on the left (black areas indicate defective parts of the field).

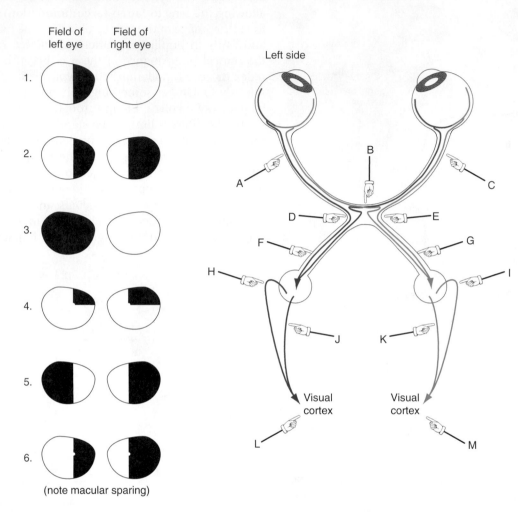

(note macular sparing)

7. Lateral interactions in the inner plexiform layer are mediated by
   a. horizontal cells.
   b. amacrine cells.
   c. bipolar cells.
   d. ganglion cells.
8. Relative to the representation of the fovea in the visual field, the blind spot is
   a. medial.
   b. lateral.
   c. superior.
   d. inferior.
9. Our color vision is best for images that fall on the
   a. fovea.
   b. region of the retina surrounding the fovea.
   c. peripheral retina.

10. Right superior homonymous quadrantanopia could be caused by damage to the
    a. sublenticular part of the right internal capsule.
    b. retrolenticular part of the right internal capsule.
    c. sublenticular part of the left internal capsule.
    d. retrolenticular part of the left internal capsule.
11. The representation of the left half of each fovea is located
    a. posteriorly in the right occipital lobe.
    b. posteriorly in the left occipital lobe.
    c. anteriorly on the medial surface of the right occipital lobe.
    d. anteriorly on the medial surface of the left occipital lobe.

Study Questions—(cont'd)

12. A large pupil that does not respond to light shone in either eye could be the result of damage to the
    a. contralateral lateral horn of the spinal cord.
    b. ipsilateral oculomotor nerve.
    c. ipsilateral optic nerve.
    d. either b or c.
    e. any of the above.

13. A person who suffers from congenital absence of retinal rods would have little difficulty in seeing the picture on a color television but would have great difficulty in seeing the picture on a black-and-white television.
    a. True
    b. False

14. Bilateral damage to the occipital lobes would abolish
    a. the pupillary light reflex.
    b. the near reflex.
    c. both reflexes.
    d. neither reflex.

15. Phototransduction in rods involves
    a. activation of an electrogenic sodium-potassium pump.
    b. activation of an enzyme that degrades cGMP.
    c. opening of cGMP-gated chloride channels.
    d. opening of cGMP-gated potassium channels.
    e. opening of photosensitive sodium channels.

Overview of Motor Systems

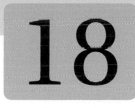

The firing rates of our motor neurons, and therefore the states of contraction of our muscles, are determined by multiple influences. Simple **reflex arcs** like the stretch reflex and more complex **motor programs** like the basic pattern generator for walking are built into the spinal cord and brainstem. These reflex arcs and motor programs, as well as the motor neurons themselves, are in turn influenced by various **descending pathways**. Finally, activity in the descending pathways is modulated by other cortical areas, the basal ganglia (see Chapter 19), and the cerebellum (see Chapter 20).

Each Lower Motor Neuron Innervates a Group of Muscle Fibers, Forming a Motor Unit

Each **lower motor neuron** innervates a fraction of the muscle fibers in one muscle. The combination of a lower motor neuron and all the muscle fibers it innervates is a **motor unit** (Fig. 18-1). Although there is a range of motor unit sizes in every muscle, their average size varies in a predictable way—those involving finely controlled muscles (e.g., extraocular muscles) contain very few muscle fibers, and those involving less finely controlled muscles may have hundreds of muscle fibers.

Lower Motor Neurons Are Arranged Systematically

The cell bodies of lower motor neurons are arranged systematically in the anterior horn (just as things like body parts and retinal areas are represented systematically in pathways and cortical areas). At any given spinal level, motor neurons for more proximal muscles are located medial to those for more distal muscles, and motor neurons for flexors are located dorsal to those for extensors (Fig. 18-2).

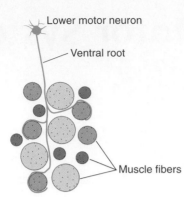

Figure 18-1   A single motor unit.

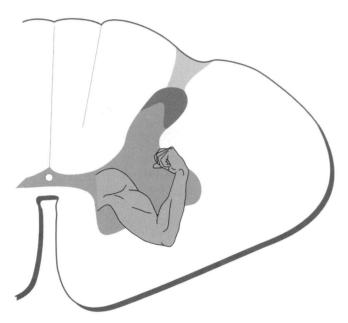

Figure 18-2   Arrangement of lower motor neurons in the anterior horn, using C8 as an example.

There Are Three Kinds of Muscle Fibers and Three Kinds of Motor Units

We use most muscles for multiple purposes that require different forces of contraction, from relatively weak contractions used in holding positions for long periods of time (e.g., standing) to powerful contractions that cannot be sustained for very long (e.g., sprinting, jumping). Corresponding to this, there are three different kinds of muscle fibers: slow fibers (**S**) that produce little force but do not fatigue much, fast fibers (**FF**) that produce a lot of force but fatigue quickly, and intermediate fibers (**FR**) with intermediate properties. All the muscle fibers innervated by a given motor neuron are of the same type, so there are also three kinds of motor units (Table 18-1).

Motor Units Are Recruited in Order of Size

If you were designing a motor-control system, you would probably set it up so that increments of force produced

Table 18-1	Motor unit types		
Type	Force	Fatigability	Recruitment Order
S	Small	Low	Early
FR	Intermediate	Intermediate	Middle
FF	Large	High	Late

by muscles were proportional in some way to the force already present—for example, making each increase in force 1% of the force already being produced by that muscle. That would make it easier to have fine control of movement. (Consider one alternative, that of having the increments be a fixed *amount* of force. The result would be adding a relatively big twitch to weak contractions and a trivial increase to strong contractions.) In fact, this proportional addition of force happens automatically because the size of the cell body of a lower motor neuron is proportional to the kind and number of muscle fibers in its motor unit (THB6 Figures 18-5 and 18-6, p. 460). It takes less synaptic input to bring a small neuron to threshold, so as upper motor neurons increase their firing frequency, motor units are recruited in order of the amount of force they produce. This **size principle** ensures the smooth gradation of muscle contraction.

Motor Control Systems Involve Both Hierarchical and Parallel Connections

Key Concepts

Reflex and motor program connections provide some of the inputs to lower motor neurons.
Upper motor neurons control lower motor neurons both directly and indirectly.
Association cortex, the cerebellum, and the basal ganglia modulate motor cortex.

The firing rates of lower motor neurons are influenced most directly by local connections and by inputs descending from more rostral levels of the CNS (i.e., **upper motor neurons**). Local connections include those that mediate simple reflexes, as well as those of **central pattern generators** or motor programs, connections that provide the basic timing signals for rhythmic activities like walking and breathing. Parallel descending inputs from several sources influence movement both directly, by synapsing on lower motor neurons, and indirectly, by synapsing on the interneurons of reflex circuits and motor programs (Fig. 18-3). The principal sources of descending inputs are the cerebral cortex (**corticospinal**

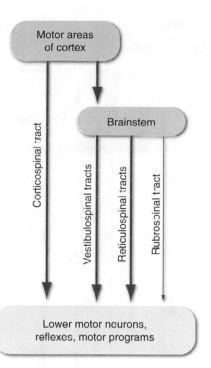

Figure 18-3   Major descending influences on lower motor neurons.

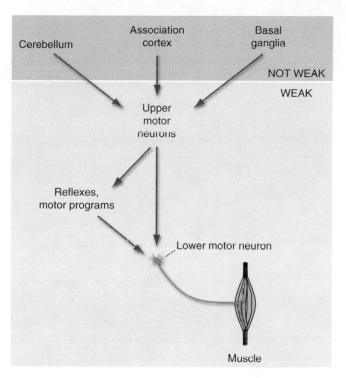

Figure 18-4   Overview of the involvement of the cerebellum, basal ganglia, and association cortex in motor control.

tract), vestibular nuclei (**vestibulospinal tracts**), and reticular formation (**reticulospinal tracts**); there is also a descending projection from the red nucleus (**rubrospinal tract**), but this is small and relatively unimportant in humans.

The **basal ganglia**, **cerebellum**, and certain areas of **association cortex** are also important in the production of movement but have little or no direct access to lower motor neurons (Fig.18-4). Rather, they affect movement by modulating the activity of upper motor neurons, particularly those in the cerebral cortex. This has important clinical consequences. Damage to motor cortex, lower motor neurons, or muscle results in weakness. In contrast, damage to the basal ganglia, cerebellum, or movement-related association cortex typically causes a variety of movement abnormalities (e.g., incoordination, involuntary movements), but not prominent weakness, because both upper and lower motor neurons are still intact.

The Corticospinal Tract Has Multiple Origins and Terminations

The principal pathway mediating voluntary movement is the corticospinal tract, a direct projection from cerebral cortex to spinal cord (together with a similar **corticobulbar tract** from cerebral cortex to cranial nerve motor nuclei). Corticospinal fibers originate from several adjacent cortical areas (see next section) and descend

through the internal capsule, cerebral peduncle, basal pons, and the medullary **pyramid** of each side. Most of these fibers then cross the midline in the **pyramidal decussation** to form the **lateral corticospinal tract** (the few uncrossed fibers form the **anterior corticospinal tract**).

Destruction of the corticospinal tract does not cause total paralysis, so there must be other descending pathways through which movements can be initiated. The major alternative is a collection of reticulospinal fibers from the brainstem reticular formation to the spinal cord. In addition, vestibulospinal tracts mediate postural adjustments and the small rubrospinal tract assists in the control of distal muscles. The rubrospinal tract, like the corticospinal tract, crosses the midline before terminating. Reticulospinal projections are bilateral, and vestibulospinal projections are mostly uncrossed.

Corticospinal Axons Arise in Multiple Cortical Areas

Key Concept

Motor cortex projects to both the spinal cord and the brainstem.

Corticospinal fibers originate from cortical areas near the central sulcus (Fig. 18-5). Many arise in **primary**

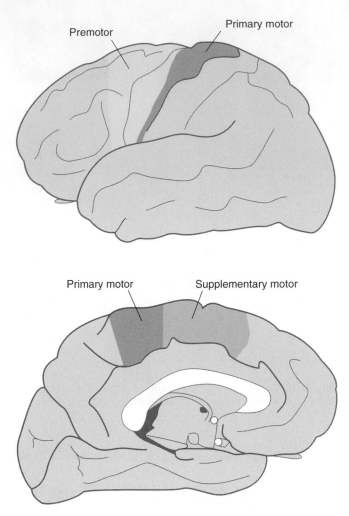

Figure 18-5 Principal motor areas of cerebral cortex.

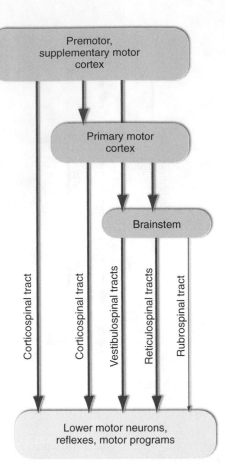

Figure 18-6 Projections of motor areas of cerebral cortex.

motor cortex in the precentral gyrus and in **premotor cortex**, just anterior to primary motor cortex. Both areas are arranged somatotopically: Neurons projecting to cranial nerve motor neurons are most ventral, those projecting to leg motor neurons are near the top of the central sulcus, and those projecting to arm and hand motor neurons are in between. Particularly large areas are devoted to the hand and mouth. In addition, some corticospinal fibers arise in the **supplementary motor area** on the medial surface of the hemisphere and others arise in the postcentral gyrus (i.e., somatosensory cortex).

Corticospinal Input Is Essential for Only Some Movements

The outputs of these cortical areas provide another example of the serial-parallel connections characteristic of the motor system (Fig. 18-6). The premotor and supplementary motor areas project to primary motor cortex, as well as projecting to the spinal cord in parallel with corticospinal fibers from primary motor cortex. In addi-

tion, all three cortical areas project not only to the spinal cord but also to brainstem sites such as the reticular formation. One consequence is that damage to motor areas of the cortex has effects (described shortly) significantly different from those following damage confined specifically to corticospinal axons, for example in the pyramid. Damage restricted to the corticospinal tract spares movements mediated by things like the reticulospinal tracts and motor programs; most severely affected are skilled, dexterous movements, notably in primates the ability to use fingers individually.

Upper Motor Neuron Damage Causes a Distinctive Syndrome

Upper motor neurons are most commonly damaged in strokes and other cortical lesions that affect corticospinal (and corticobulbar) neurons. The result is **spastic hemiparesis**, in which the contralateral side of the body is weak, stretch reflexes are increased, and muscle tone is increased. The flexors of the upper extremity and extensors of the lower extremity are particularly affected. **Babinski's sign** (dorsiflexion of the big toe and fanning of the others in response to firmly stroking the sole of the foot) is also present on the side contralateral to the lesion, and **clonus** (rhythmic contractions in response to maintained muscle stretch) may be seen. The increased tone collapses abruptly in response to strong efforts to overcome it (**clasp-knife response**).

Spastic hemiparesis is the result of massive disruption of the output from motor areas of the cortex, including outputs to the brainstem reticular formation. Hence, it can result from damage to the cerebral cortex, the posterior limb of the internal capsule, or the spinal cord (where corticospinal and other descending fibers are intermingled to some extent). On the other hand, damage only to primary motor cortex or selective damage to the corticospinal fibers in the pyramid causes weakness and Babinski's sign, but not marked spasticity.

Spasticity is very different from the results of lower motor neuron damage. Lower motor neuron disease is also accompanied by weakness, but in this case reflexes and tone are diminished. In addition, the weak muscles **fasciculate** and **atrophy**.

There Are Upper Motor Neurons for Cranial Nerve Motor Nuclei

Axons of the upper motor neurons for cranial nerve motor nuclei form the corticobulbar tract (Fig. 18-7). These fibers mostly accompany the corticospinal tract until they reach the level of the nuclei in which they terminate. In contrast to corticospinal fibers, however, they are distributed bilaterally to a great extent. The result is that, with one major exception, corticobulbar damage on one side does not cause lasting contralateral weakness of muscles innervated by cranial nerves. The major exception is the muscles of the lower face, whose motor neurons are innervated predominantly by contralateral cerebral cortex, with the result that corticobulbar damage on one side causes contralateral weakness of only the lower face (see Fig. 12-9). In addition, the trigeminal and hypoglossal nuclei receive more crossed than uncrossed fibers in most individuals, and corticobulbar damage can result in slight and usually transient weakness of the contralateral jaw or tongue.

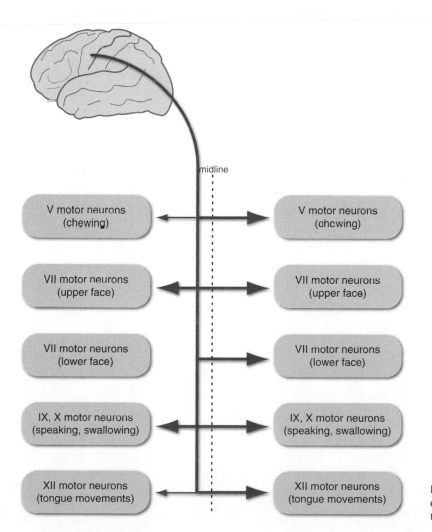

Figure 18-7   Corticobulbar tract. The thickness of each line indicates the relative magnitude of the projection.

Study Questions

1. A 72-year-old theremin tuner with a history of cardiovascular disease had the sudden onset of confusion, during which her left arm and leg became weak. The weakness was most likely due to damage to which of the following?
   a. left cerebellar hemisphere.
   b. right inferior frontal gyrus.
   c. right internal capsule.
   d. right lenticular nucleus.
   e. right superior parietal lobule.

2. Descending influences on spinal cord motor neurons include all of the following *except*
   a. crossed projections from the red nucleus.
   b. crossed projections from the ventral lateral (VL) nucleus of the thalamus.
   c. bilateral reticulospinal projections.
   d. uncrossed projections from the vestibular nuclei to antigravity muscles.

3. Moving superiorly from the lateral sulcus, the order of representation of body parts in primary motor cortex is
   a. leg, arm, head.
   b. arm, leg, head.
   c. arm, head, leg.
   d. leg, head, arm.
   e. head, arm, leg.

4. The supplementary motor area is located
   a. on the medial surface of the hemisphere, anterior to primary motor cortex.
   b. on the medial surface of the hemisphere, posterior to primary motor cortex.
   c. on the lateral surface of the hemisphere, anterior to primary motor cortex.
   d. in the parietal lobe, posterior to somatosensory cortex.
   e. on the lateral surface of the hemisphere, anterior to premotor cortex.

5. Upper motor neuron disease and lower motor neuron disease are similar in that in both conditions
   a. stretch reflexes are diminished.
   b. muscles fasciculate and atrophy.
   c. the flexors of the upper extremity are affected more than the extensors.
   d. Babinski's sign is present.
   e. none of the above.

6. Spasticity on the right would be likely after damage to the
   a. left frontal lobe.
   b. posterior limb of the left internal capsule.
   c. left lateral funiculus of the spinal cord.
   d. either a or b.
   e. any of the above.

7. Damage to motor cortex on one side typically causes the most contralateral weakness when
   a. speaking.
   b. swallowing.
   c. raising eyebrows.
   d. smiling.

8. As the biceps is contracted more and more forcefully, the order in which motor units are recruited is
   a. FF, FR, S.
   b. FF, S, FR.
   c. FR, FF, S.
   d. FR, S, FF.
   e. S, FF, FR.
   f. S, FR, FF.

Basal Ganglia

Historically, the basal ganglia have been considered as major components of the motor system. In fact, they have a much broader role than that and are probably involved to some extent in most forebrain functions. However, their relationship to movement is their best understood aspect, and that is what shows up clinically in disorders like Parkinson's disease and Huntington's disease. The interrelationships of the basal ganglia and motor areas of the cerebral cortex are emphasized in this chapter, but you should keep in mind that the basal ganglia have extensive connections, similar in principle and parallel in detail, with most other areas of the cerebral cortex.

The Basal Ganglia Include Five Major Nuclei

Key Concepts

The striatum and globus pallidus are the major forebrain components of the basal ganglia.

The substantia nigra and subthalamic nucleus are interconnected with the striatum and globus pallidus.

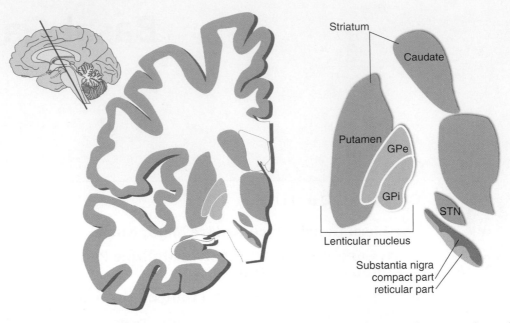

Figure 19-1   Major components of the basal ganglia, and terminology used to refer to them. Nucleus accumbens, the third component of the striatum, lies anterior to this plane of section. *GPe*, External segment of the globus pallidus; *GPi*, internal segment of the globus pallidus; *STN*, subthalamic nucleus.

The meaning of the term "basal ganglia" has changed over the years, but most folks would now agree that there are five major structures on the list: the **caudate nucleus**, **putamen**, **globus pallidus**, **substantia nigra**, and **subthalamic nucleus** (Fig. 19-1). The caudate nucleus and putamen have similar but parallel connections and are referred to in combination as the **striatum**. The putamen and globus pallidus have very different connections but are physically stuck together; in combination, they are referred to as the **lenticular nucleus** (from the Latin word for "lentil").

The terms **strio-** and **-striate** are used to refer to fibers coming from or going to the striatum; for example, corticostriate fibers start in the cerebral cortex and end in the caudate nucleus or putamen. Similarly, the terms **pallido-** and **-pallidal**, **nigro-** and **-nigral**, and **subthalamo-** and **-subthalamic** are used to refer to fibers coming from or going to the globus pallidus, the substantia nigra, or the subthalamic nucleus.

The caudate nucleus parallels the lateral ventricle, having an enlarged **head** in the wall of the anterior horn, a smaller **body** adjacent to the body of the ventricle, and a still smaller **tail** adjacent to the inferior horn.

The caudate nucleus and putamen merge with each other anteriorly at the base of the septum pellucidum; the area of fusion is **nucleus accumbens**, now recognized as a third division of the striatum.

The lenticular nucleus (putamen + globus pallidus) underlies the insula and is shaped like a wedge cut from a sphere (THB6 Figures 19-1 and 19-2, pp. 475 and 476). The globus pallidus is the more medial, tapering part of the wedge, extending toward the interventricular foramen and thalamus; it has two parts with distinctive connections, an **external segment** (**GPe**) adjacent to the putamen and an **internal segment** (**GPi**) closer to the thalamus.

The substantia nigra is mostly located in the rostral midbrain, between the cerebral peduncle and the red nucleus; part of it extends rostrally just into the diencephalon. The substantia nigra is another two-part structure. The **compact part** (**SNc**), closer to the red nucleus, contains the pigmented, dopaminergic neurons for which the substantia nigra was named; the **reticular part** (**SNr**), adjacent to the cerebral peduncle, is in effect a displaced piece of GPi.

The subthalamic nucleus, as its name implies, is located inferior to the thalamus, just above the most rostral part of the substantia nigra.

Basal Ganglia Circuitry Involves Multiple Parallel Loops That Modulate Cortical Output

Key Concept

Afferents from the cortex reach the striatum and subthalamic nucleus; efferents leave from the globus pallidus and substantia nigra.

How does damage to the basal ganglia cause movement (and other) disorders? For the most part, we know only the broad outlines of an answer, but there is one basic fact to keep in mind: The basal ganglia have no major outputs to lower motor neurons. Instead, they work primarily by influencing what comes out of the cerebral cortex.

The striatum is, in a sense, the major input part of the basal ganglia, collecting excitatory (glutamate) inputs from large cortical areas (different areas for different parts of the striatum). GPi and SNr are the principal output structures, sending inhibitory (GABA) projections to the thalamus, which in turn projects back to a restricted portion of this large cortical area (Fig. 19-2). Because thalamocortical projections are excitatory, the globus pallidus is in a position to suppress or facilitate cortical activity by way of varying patterns of inhibition in the thalamus; the balance of excitatory and inhibitory connections interposed between the striatum and GPi/SNr helps determine the pattern. For example, inhibiting an inhibitory GPi neuron could have the same net effect on the thalamus as increasing excitatory inputs to the same part of the thalamus (Fig. 19-3).

All these structures, and most of their interconnections, are in one cerebral hemisphere, so damage to any of them results in contralateral deficits.

Although the cortex-striatum-globus pallidus-thalamus-cortex pathway is commonly drawn as a single loop, it is actually a system of parallel, overlapping loops, each wired up according to the same principles (Fig. 19-4). So the caudate nucleus, for example, receives its inputs from a different widespread area of the cortex than does the putamen and influences its own part of the globus pallidus, which in turn projects to its own part of the thalamus and its own restricted cortical area.

The putamen subsystem is the part most directly involved in movement disorders. Its inputs come from

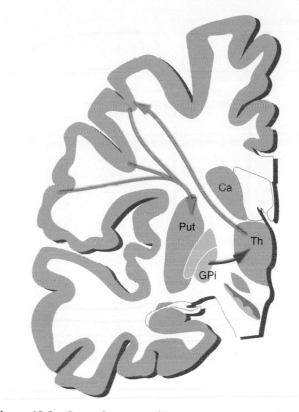

Figure 19-2 General pattern of input-output connections of the basal ganglia. The putamen (Put) is shown as an example of the striatum; the caudate nucleus (Ca) and nucleus accumbens (not in this plane of section) have similar connections, but with different areas of cortex and different parts of GPi and the thalamus (Th). Excitatory connections are shown in green, inhibitory connections in red.

the motor and somatosensory areas flanking the central sulcus. Its outputs reach motor areas of cortex (particularly the **supplementary motor area**) by way of the ventral lateral and ventral anterior nuclei of the thalamus (VL and VA). This set of connections is consistent

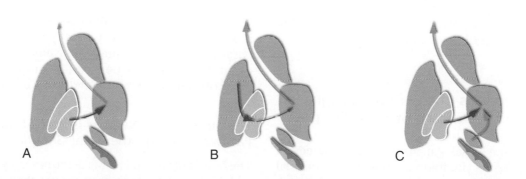

Figure 19-3 An illustration of the way in which activity in some part of the nervous system can be enhanced by either inhibition or excitation of some other part of the nervous system. Baseline levels of activity in thalamocortical neurons (**A**) could be enhanced either by inhibiting inhibition of the thalamus (**B**) or by increasing excitatory inputs to the thalamus (**C**). Excitatory connections are shown in green, inhibitory connections in red.

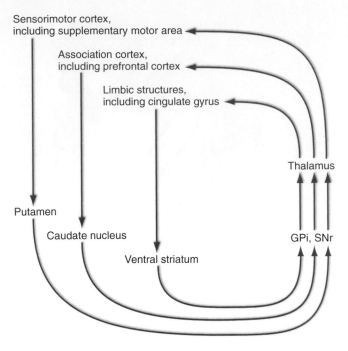

Figure 19-4 Parallel loops through the basal ganglia.

The Cerebral Cortex, Substantia Nigra, and Thalamus Project to the Striatum

> ### Key Concepts
>
> Part of the substantia nigra modulates the output of the striatum and other parts of the basal ganglia.
> Different parts of the striatum are involved in movement, cognition, and affect.
> The striatum projects to the globus pallidus and substantia nigra.
> The external segment of the globus pallidus distributes inhibitory signals within the basal ganglia.

Although inputs from the cerebral cortex predominate, modulatory **dopaminergic** projections from SNc (to the caudate and putamen) and from the **ventral tegmental area** (to the ventral striatum) are a second important category of striatal inputs; disruption of these connections causes **Parkinson's disease**. Some **intralaminar nuclei** also project to the striatum, but little is known of the significance of these connections.

The Internal Segment of the Globus Pallidus and the Reticular Part of the Substantia Nigra Provide the Output from the Basal Ganglia

Different parts of the striatum project to particular parts of the globus pallidus (both segments) and SNr. GPe sends inhibitory projections to most other parts of the basal ganglia, but GPi and SNr provide the major outputs from the basal ganglia. Pallidal output fibers (from GPi) reach the thalamus through two bundles (THB6 Figure 19-15, p. 485). The **ansa lenticularis** hooks around the medial edge of the internal capsule. The **lenticular fasciculus** passes directly through the internal capsule. The two bundles join cerebellar output fibers beneath the thalamus and form the **thalamic fasciculus**, which then enters the thalamus.

The cortex-striatum-GPi/SNr-thalamus-cortex loop is often considered to be a **direct pathway** through the basal ganglia that facilitates movement (Fig. 19-5), a circuit whose malfunction partially explains the slow, diminished movements of Parkinson's disease.

The Subthalamic Nucleus Is Part of an Indirect Pathway through the Basal Ganglia

The output of GPi and SNr is determined by the balance of inhibitory and excitatory inputs they receive. The striatum is a major source of inhibitory inputs. The subthalamic nucleus, on the other hand, provides a power-

with the notion that the putamen and supplementary motor area are somehow involved in planning or initiating voluntary movements.

The caudate nucleus, in contrast, is more involved in cognitive functions, although less is known about how this involvement shows up in our day-to-day activities. Caudate inputs come from widespread **association areas** of the cerebral cortex; caudate outputs, by way of VA and the dorsomedial nucleus (DM), reach prefrontal cortex. So the anatomical connections are appropriate for an involvement of the caudate in cognitive functions.

Finally, nucleus accumbens and adjacent striatal areas (collectively called the **ventral striatum**) receive inputs from limbic structures and project, by way of part of the globus pallidus and thalamus, back to **limbic cortex** (described in Chapter 23).

Interconnections of the Basal Ganglia Determine the Pattern of Their Outputs

Processing in the basal ganglia is largely based on fluctuating levels of inhibition. Striatal and pallidal neurons all use GABA as a transmitter; the subthalamic nucleus is the only major source of excitatory (glutamate) projections.

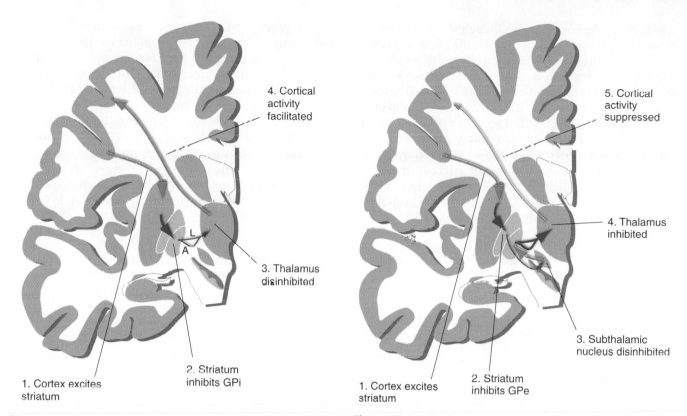

4. Cortical
activity
facilitated

L
A

3. Thalamus
disinhibited

1. Cortex excites
striatum

2. Striatum
inhibits GPi

5. Cortical
activity
suppressed

4. Thalamus
inhibited

3. Subthalamic
nucleus disinhibited

1. Cortex excites
striatum

2. Striatum
inhibits GPe

Figure 19-5 The "direct pathway" through the basal ganglia. *A,* Ansa lenticularis; *L,* lenticular fasciculus. Excitatory connections are shown in green, inhibitory connections in red.

Figure 19-6 The "indirect pathway" through the basal ganglia. Excitatory connections are shown in green, inhibitory connections in red.

ful excitatory input. The subthalamic nucleus is often considered to be part of an **indirect pathway** through the basal ganglia (Fig. 19-6), one that has just the opposite effect on thalamic activity as the direct pathway. According to one model of basal ganglia function, the balance of activity in the direct and indirect pathways helps to determine which cortical activities are facilitated and which are suppressed. The fibers that travel back and forth between the subthalamic nucleus and the globus pallidus penetrate the internal capsule as small bundles that are collectively called the **subthalamic fasciculus** (THB6 Figure 19-16, p. 486).

Perforating Branches from the Circle of Willis Supply the Basal Ganglia

Like other deep cerebral structures, the basal ganglia are supplied by perforating branches from the circle of Willis; the pattern is predictable from the anterior-posterior layout of components of the basal ganglia. The substantia nigra and subthalamic nucleus are in or near the midbrain, so they are supplied by branches from posterior parts of the circle (i.e., from the posterior

cerebral and posterior communicating arteries). The lenticular nucleus, a little farther anterior, is supplied by the anterior choroidal artery and branches of the middle cerebral artery. Finally, anterior cerebral branches help supply nucleus accumbens and the head of the caudate nucleus.

Many Basal Ganglia Disorders Result in Abnormalities of Movement

Key Concept

Anatomical and neurochemical properties of the basal ganglia suggest effective treatments for disorders.

The best-known basal ganglia disorders are characterized by a combination of **positive** and **negative signs**—positive signs being involuntary muscle contractions in various patterns and negative signs being difficulty producing muscle contraction. Parkinson's disease is the classic example. Positive signs include a **resting tremor**, especially pronounced in the hands, and a general increase in tone in all muscles, referred to as **rigidity**. Negative signs include slow movements (**bradykinesia**) and reduced numbers of movements (**hypokinesia** or **akinesia**). There's no particular change in strength or reflexes. Other basal ganglia disorders can be accompanied by different kinds of involuntary movements that fall into three general categories: rapid movements called **chorea**; slow, writhing movements called **athetosis**; and flailing movements of entire limbs, called **ballism**. In some disorders, tone is increased even more than in Parkinson's; in others, it is decreased.

Many symptoms of basal ganglia disorders seem consistent with the direct-indirect circuit model (THB6 Figure 19-21, p. 490). For example, disruption of the dopaminergic projection from the substantia nigra to the striatum, the cause of Parkinson's disease, would be expected to increase GPi/SNr output and suppress movement. Also, damaging the subthalamic nucleus would disable the indirect pathway and in fact causes ballism on the contralateral side (i.e., contralateral **hemiballismus**). However, other observations are incompatible and make it seem likely that the direct-indirect circuit model is at best a partial explanation.

Study Questions

1. A 39-year-old handball hustler noticed the abrupt onset of involuntary movements of his right side. His right arm and leg would make large, violent, flailing movements that interfered with his game. The most likely site of damage was his
   a. left substantia nigra.
   b. right substantia nigra.
   c. left globus pallidus.
   d. right globus pallidus.
   e. left subthalamic nucleus.
   f. right subthalamic nucleus.
2. The term "strionigral fibers" could be used to refer to fibers that project from the
   a. caudate nucleus to the substantia nigra.
   b. substantia nigra to the putamen.
   c. subthalamic nucleus to the substantia nigra.
   d. globus pallidus to the substantia nigra.
3. The major source of inputs to the caudate nucleus is
   a. the globus pallidus.
   b. the subthalamic nucleus.
   c. the putamen.
   d. association areas of the cortex, like prefrontal cortex.
   e. motor and somatosensory cortex.
4. The major circuit through which the basal ganglia affect the cerebral cortex involves a projection from the
   a. globus pallidus to the thalamus.
   b. globus pallidus to the substantia nigra.
   c. striatum to the thalamus.
   d. striatum to the cerebral cortex.
   e. globus pallidus to the cerebral cortex.
5. Spasticity and parkinsonian rigidity are similar in that in both conditions there is
   a. weakness.
   b. increased stretch reflexes.
   c. increased biceps tone.
   d. tremor at rest.
   e. none of the above.
6. The basal ganglia include all of the following *except* the
   a. globus pallidus.
   b. putamen.
   c. substantia nigra.
   d. thalamus.
   e. subthalamic nucleus.

Answer questions 7-11 using the following diagram. Each question may have multiple answers, and each letter can be used more than once.

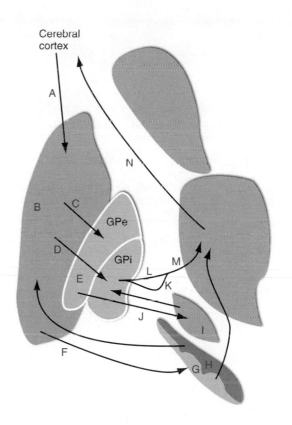

7. Thalamic fasciculus.
8. Subthalamic nucleus.
9. Location of neuronal cell bodies that use dopamine as a neurotransmitter.
10. Location of neuronal cell bodies that use GABA as a neurotransmitter.
11. Location of neuronal cell bodies that use glutamate as a neurotransmitter.

Cerebellum

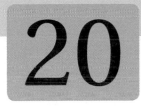

The cerebellum helps coordinate movement by sampling most kinds of sensory information, comparing current movements with intended movements, and issuing planning or correcting signals. The comparisons are made in a uniform, precisely organized, cerebellar cortex and the planning or correcting signals are issued through a set of deep cerebellar nuclei. Because its output is concerned with coordination of movement and not with perception, cerebellar lesions cause incoordination but no sensory changes.

The Cerebellum Can Be Divided into Transverse and Longitudinal Zones

Key Concepts

Transverse fissures divide the cerebellum into lobes.
Functional connections divide the cerebellum into longitudinal zones.

In a gross anatomical sense, the **primary fissure** divides the bulk of the cerebellum into **anterior** and **posterior lobes**, and another deep fissure separates the **flocculus** and **nodulus** (together forming the **flocculonodular lobe**) from the **body** of the cerebellum (Fig. 20-1). Assorted exotic names are sometimes applied to various parts of the anterior and posterior lobes, but most are of limited clinical utility. One worth remembering is the **tonsil**, the part of the posterior lobe nearest to the flocculus (THB6 Figure 20-2D, p. 496). The tonsil is one of the most inferior parts of the cerebellum, and expanding masses in the posterior fossa can cause it to herniate through the foramen magnum, compressing the medulla (THB6 Figure 4-19D, p. 96).

In terms of connections and functions, however, it is more useful to divide each half of the cerebellum into three longitudinal zones—a midline **vermis** and a **hemisphere** with a **medial** and a larger **lateral** part. The vermis is involved in coordination of trunk movements. The medial and lateral parts of the hemisphere are both involved in ipsilateral limb movements, but in different ways.

Deep Nuclei Are Embedded in the Cerebellar White Matter

The fundamental building plan of the cerebellum as a whole involves afferents that reach the cerebellar cortex, which in turn projects to deep nuclei embedded in the cerebellar white matter. The deep nuclei then give rise to the output of the cerebellum. There are a series of

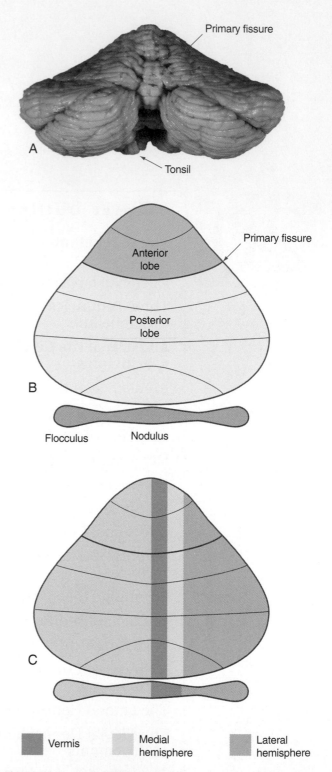

Figure 20-1 A posterior view of the cerebellum (**A**), and two similar cartoon views showing its division transversely into lobes (**B**) and longitudinally into functional zones (**C**). The cartoon view is as though you were looking from behind at a cerebellum that had been flattened out so that all of its parts could be seen.

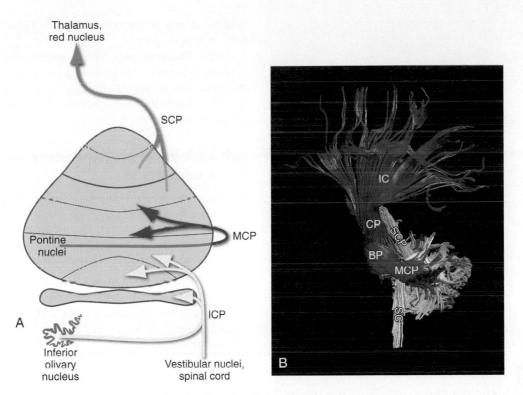

Figure 20-2 **A**, Contents of the cerebellar peduncles. For simplicity, the inferior and superior peduncles are shown as being entirely afferent and efferent; each actually contains a smaller number of fibers traveling in the opposite direction. *ICP*, Inferior cerebellar peduncle; *MCP*, middle cerebellar peduncle; *SCP*, superior cerebellar peduncle. **B**, A beautiful diffusion tensor image (see THB6 Box 5-1, p. 118) of the cerebellar peduncles, seen from the left side. Fibers from widespread cortical areas descend through the internal capsule (IC), funnel into the cerebral peduncle (CP), and reach pontine nuclei in the basal pons (BP); pontine nuclei then project to the contralateral half of the cerebellum through the middle cerebellar peduncle (MCP). Spinocerebellar fibers (SC) enter the cerebellum through the inferior cerebellar peduncle. Finally, cerebellar efferents leave through the superior cerebellar peduncle (SCP). Shorter fibers that interconnect different parts of the cerebellum are shown in blue. *(Modified from Catani M et al: Altered cerebellar feedback projections in Asperger syndrome. NeuroImage 41:1184, 2008. Thanks to Dr. Marco Catani.)*

three deep nuclei on each side, arranged in a medial to lateral array: the **fastigial** (most medial), **interposed**, and **dentate** (most lateral) **nuclei** (THB6 Figure 20-7, p. 501).

Three Peduncles Convey the Input and Output of Each Half of the Cerebellum

Three peduncles containing the cerebellar afferents and efferents attach the cerebellum to the brainstem (Fig. 20-2). The **superior cerebellar peduncle** is the major output route from its side of the cerebellum, carrying all the efferents from the dentate and interposed nuclei and some of the efferents from the fastigial nucleus. The **middle cerebellar peduncle** is the input route for information from the cerebral cortex, carrying the fibers from contralateral **pontine nuclei**. By elimination then, the **inferior cerebellar peduncle** is a complex bundle, carrying most of the remaining cerebellar afferents (including **climbing fibers**, as described a little later), as well as the remaining cerebellar efferents.

All Parts of the Cerebellum Share Common Organizational Principles

All parts of the cerebellum have a cortex with the same structure and use the same basic circuitry (Fig. 20-3; inputs → cortex → deep nuclei → outputs). This suggests that all parts of the cerebellum perform the same basic (still mysterious) operation, and that the functional differences among different cerebellar regions are simply reflections of different input sources and output targets.

Inputs Reach the Cerebellar Cortex as Mossy and Climbing Fibers

Afferents reach the cerebellar cortex in two forms: **mossy fibers** and **climbing fibers** (Fig. 20-4). Climbing fibers, all from the contralateral **inferior olivary nucleus**, end directly on **Purkinje cells**, which provide the output from cerebellar cortex. Mossy fibers, in contrast, come

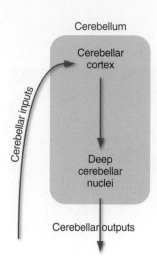

Figure 20-3 General pattern of cerebellar inputs and outputs.

from many other places and end on the tiny **granule cells** of the cerebellar cortex; these in turn issue **parallel fibers** that synapse on Purkinje cells. Although mossy fibers arise on both sides of the CNS, those reaching one side of the cerebellum carry information related to the

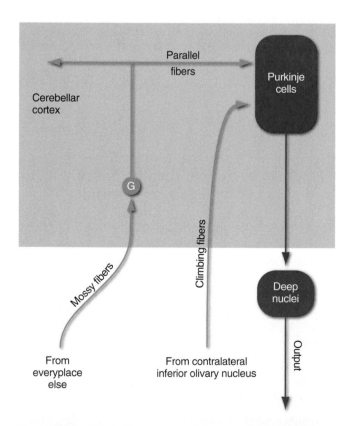

Figure 20-4 Cerebellar cortex and deep nuclei. Excitatory connections are shown in green, inhibitory connections in red. Projections from the deep nuclei are shown in a third color because, although most are excitatory, some are inhibitory. *G,* Granule cells.

ipsilateral side of the body (e.g., see Figs. 20-6 and 20-7 later in this chapter).

Some Purkinje cell axons project directly to the vestibular nuclei. Except for these, however, the entire Purkinje cell output is directed to the deep cerebellar nuclei, which in turn provide the output from the cerebellum.

Purkinje Cells of the Cerebellar Cortex Project to the Deep Nuclei

The flocculonodular lobe is primarily concerned with vestibular function (posture and eye movements), and most of its output is directed to the vestibular nuclei either directly or indirectly. The three longitudinal zones of the remainder of the cerebellum direct their outputs to three deep nuclei arranged in a corresponding medial-to-lateral array (Fig. 20-5): vermis → fastigial nucleus, medial hemisphere → interposed (globose + emboliform) nucleus, and lateral hemisphere → dentate nucleus.

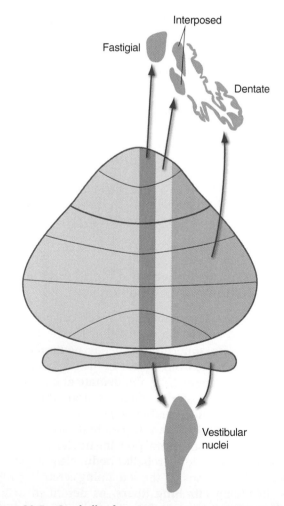

Figure 20-5 Cerebellar functional zones and deep nuclei.

One Side of the Cerebellum Affects the Ipsilateral Side of the Body

Each fastigial nucleus, relaying the output from the vermis, projects bilaterally to the reticular formation and vestibular nuclei. However, the medial hemisphere/interposed nucleus and lateral hemisphere/dentate nucleus systems of each side are connected so that they help control ipsilateral limbs. What this means is that even though there are lots of midline crossings in cerebellar circuitry, they all fit together so that one side of the cerebellum affects ipsilateral limbs. For example, cerebral cortex on one side affects contralateral limbs, so it in turn must be connected to the contralateral half of the cerebellum as well.

Details of Connections Differ Among Zones

Each functional zone of the cerebellum is connected not only with a particular output nucleus, but also with a distinctive set of inputs (Fig. 20-6). The flocculonodular lobe primarily receives vestibular afferents. The vermis and medial hemispheres receive **spinocerebellar** inputs and inputs from motor cortex (via pontine nuclei). The lateral hemispheres receive inputs via the **pontine nuclei** from widespread cortical areas. (These are not the only inputs to these zones, but they do provide a hint about the principal function of each zone.)

Cerebellar Cortex Receives Inputs from Multiple Sources

Each bit of cerebellar cortex receives multiple inputs, but in a distinguishing pattern—climbing fibers from a particular part of the contralateral inferior olivary nucleus, mossy fibers from contralateral pontine nuclei reflecting input from a particular cortical area, and some others that are unique to that part of the cerebellar cortex.

Vestibular Inputs Reach the Flocculus and Vermis

Vestibular inputs reach the flocculonodular lobe and the vermis as well. These come both from the vestibular nuclei and also directly from the vestibular nerve.

The Spinal Cord Projects to the Vermis and Medial Hemisphere

The vermis and particularly the medial hemisphere receive overlapping mossy fiber inputs from the ipsilateral spinal cord and trigeminal nuclei (hence, the ipsilateral side of the body) and the contralateral cerebral cortex (hence, the ipsilateral side of the body once again), in a superimposed, roughly somatotopic pattern (THB6

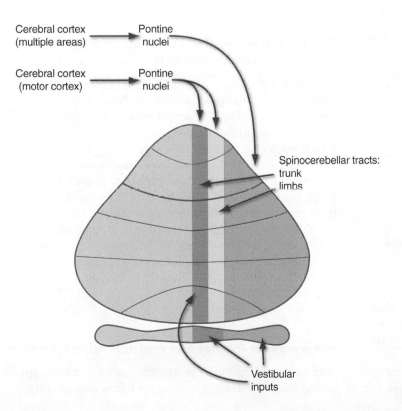

Figure 20-6 Principal sources of mossy fibers to cerebellar functional zones.

Figure 20-17, p. 510). Both spinal and cortical (mainly from motor cortex) inputs representing the limbs reach the medial hemisphere; those representing the trunk reach the vermis.

Cerebral Cortex Projects to the Cerebellum by Way of Pontine Nuclei

Both the inputs and the outputs of the lateral cerebellar hemisphere emphasize the cerebral cortex. Inputs, by way of pontine nuclei, come from contralateral motor, premotor, somatosensory, and even association cortex. Things like spinocerebellar and vestibulocerebellar fibers don't reach this part of the cerebellum, again providing a hint about its function.

Climbing Fibers Arise in the Inferior Olivary Nucleus

The inferior olivary nucleus is the sole source of the climbing fibers that blanket the contralateral half of the cerebellum. The projection is topographically organized, so each small part of the inferior olivary nucleus projects to a particular small region of the cerebellar cortex.

Visual and Auditory Information Reaches the Cerebellum

The cerebellum does not use just somatosensory information to help plan and guide movement. Projections from parts of visual and auditory cortex, by way of their own subset of pontine nuclei, reach the part of the vermis that receives somatosensory information from the head.

Each Longitudinal Zone Has a Distinctive Output

Key Concepts

The vermis projects to the fastigial nucleus.
The medial and lateral parts of each hemisphere project to the interposed and dentate nuclei.

Each functional zone of cerebellar cortex has not only a distinguishing set of inputs (see Fig. 20-6), but also a distinguishing pattern of projections to the deep nuclei (see Fig. 20-5). The deep nuclei in turn have further projections that make functional sense.

The fastigial nucleus projects through the inferior cerebellar peduncle mainly to the vestibular nuclei and

reticular formation. The interposed and dentate nuclei project through the superior cerebellar peduncle, most of whose fibers cross the midline in the caudal midbrain, pass through or around the **red nucleus**, and reach VL/VA of the thalamus (Fig. 20-7). Some fibers from the interposed nucleus end in the part of the red nucleus that gives rise to the rubrospinal tract; some from the dentate nucleus reach the (much larger) part of the red nucleus that in turn projects to the inferior olivary nucleus.

Patterns of Connections Indicate the Functions of Longitudinal Zones

The distinctive patterns of connections of the different functional zones of the cerebellum are generally consistent with the kinds of deficits that follow damage to each zone.

The Lateral Hemispheres Are Involved in Planning Movements

The connections of the lateral hemispheres are dominated by a great loop from cerebral cortex, through the cerebellum, and back to motor and premotor cortex. This is the anatomical substrate for a role of the lateral hemispheres in the planning of movements, particularly learned movements that become more rapid and precise over time.

The Medial Hemispheres Are Involved in Adjusting Limb Movements

The medial parts of the cerebellar hemispheres, in contrast, are set up to compare intended movement (inputs from motor cortex) and actual movement (spinal cord sensory information). Correcting signals from the interposed nucleus then leave the cerebellum via the superior cerebellar peduncle, cross the midline in the **decussation of the superior cerebellar peduncles**, and reach the red nucleus and thalamus. **Rubrospinal** fibers then recross the midline and travel to the spinal cord. Thus the medial hemisphere of one side is related to ipsilateral limb movements. The interposed nucleus can also influence corticospinal output by means of projections through VL of the thalamus; in humans, these connections are more important functionally than the rubrospinal projection.

The Vermis Is Involved in Postural Adjustments

Vermal inputs, from the vestibular nuclei and from spinocerebellar fibers representing the trunk, are concerned

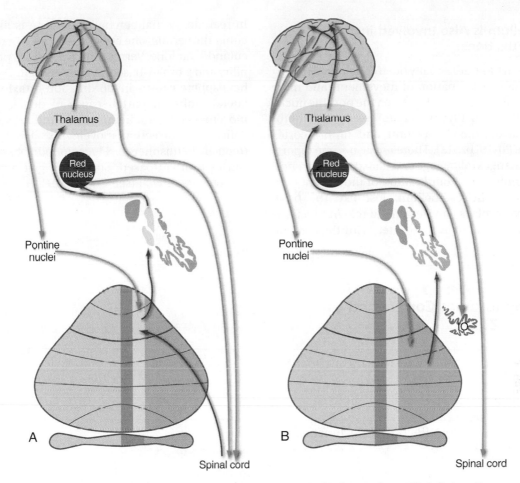

Figure 20-7 Pattern of connections of the medial (**A**) and lateral (**B**) cerebellar hemisphere. *IO*, Inferior olivary nucleus.

with the general orientation and posture of the body. Similarly, vermal outputs affect vestibulospinal and reticulospinal neurons that are related to antigravity and other proximal muscles, suggesting a role in adjusting posture and motor programs (e.g., walking).

The Flocculus and Vermis Are Involved in Eye Movements

As mentioned in Chapter 14 and again in Chapter 21, the vestibular system plays a major role in vestibuloocular and other kinds of smooth eye movements. The vestibular connections of the flocculus make it another important player in smooth eye movements (see Chapter 21). In addition, the vestibular/visual connections of the vermis enable it to play a role in the coordination of gaze shifts (see Chapter 21), just as the rest of the cerebellum is important in the coordination of movements generally.

The Cerebellum Is Involved in Motor Learning

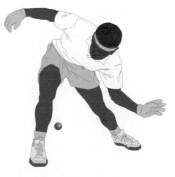

We usually think of learning in terms of facts and events, but there are actually multiple kinds of memory—we can learn not only facts, but also skills, habits, emotional associations, and even modified reflex responses. The cerebellum is involved at least in the modification of reflexes and in the acquisition of new physical skills. Although the details are not understood yet, the powerful excitatory synapses that climbing fibers make on Purkinje cells are critically involved in the changes that underlie these forms of **motor learning**.

The Cerebellum Is Also Involved in Cognitive Functions

The cerebellum has traditionally been considered important only for the coordination of movement (and more recently for motor learning). However, the pontine nuclei receive inputs not just from somatosensory and motor cortex, but also from association and limbic cortex (THB6 Figure 20-19, p. 511). There are also some reports of cognitive changes following cerebellar damage. Hence, although planning and coordination of movement is its major function, the cerebellum, just like the basal ganglia, probably plays a more general role in functions that we usually think of as associated with the cerebral cortex.

In real life, partial cerebellar damage is likely to affect either the vermis, one cerebellar hemisphere, or the flocculonodular lobe. Vermal damage causes postural instability and a broad-based, staggering gait. Damage to one hemisphere causes incoordination (**ataxia**) of the ipsilateral limbs, in part because of deficits in planning movements (lateral hemisphere) and in part because of deficits in correcting movements already under way (medial hemisphere). Flocculonodular damage also causes a broad-based, staggering gait and affects eye movements as well (see Chapter 21).

Clinical Syndromes Correspond to Functional Zones

Key Concepts

Midline damage causes postural instability.
Lateral damage causes limb ataxia.
Damage to the flocculus affects eye movements.

Study Questions

1. The axons of cerebellar granule cells are
   a. parallel fibers.
   b. mossy fibers.
   c. climbing fibers.
   d. the principal output from cerebellar cortex.
   e. figments of Jack Nolte's imagination.

2. Most of the output of the cerebellum is in the form of
   a. Purkinje cell axons.
   b. climbing fibers.
   c. axons of neurons in the deep cerebellar nuclei.
   d. mossy fibers.

3. The cortex of the cerebellar vermis projects mainly to the
   a. fastigial nucleus.
   b. dentate nucleus.
   c. interposed nucleus.
   d. vestibular nuclei.

4. The flocculonodular lobe projects mainly to the
   a. fastigial nucleus.
   b. dentate nucleus.
   c. interposed nucleus.
   d. vestibular nuclei.

5. The primary fissure of the cerebellum marks the division between the
   a. anterior and posterior lobes.
   b. anterior and flocculonodular lobes.
   c. posterior and flocculonodular lobes.
   d. vermis and the medial hemisphere.
   e. medial hemisphere and the lateral hemisphere.

6. Spinocerebellar fibers carrying information about limb position project mainly to the
   a. medial hemisphere.
   b. lateral hemisphere.
   c. vermis.

7. Information traveling from the right cerebral hemisphere to the cerebellum crosses the midline
   a. in the decussation of the superior cerebellar peduncles.
   b. on its way from the right thalamus (VL/VA) to the pons.
   c. in the pons, as pontocerebellar fibers.
   d. This information does not cross the midline.

For questions 8-10, match the fiber types in the column on the left with the cerebellar peduncles in the column on the right; each peduncle may be used more than once or not at all.

8. Climbing fibers
9. Output fibers from the interposed nucleus
10. Projections from the cerebellum to vestibular nuclei

   a. Inferior cerebellar peduncle
   b. Middle cerebellar peduncle
   c. Superior cerebellar peduncle

11. There is a small spino-olivary tract from the spinal cord to the inferior olivary nucleus. On the basis of what you know about cerebellar connections, would you expect this tract to be mostly crossed or mostly uncrossed?

Control of Eye Movements

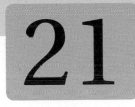

Photoreceptors throughout the animal kingdom use G protein–coupled transduction mechanisms for added sensitivity, but they pay a price in speed: Images need to stay still on the retina for a tenth of second or so at a time to be seen clearly. And for animals with a fovea (like us), images need to stay still on precisely that small part of the retina. All animals with image-forming eyes alternate between relatively brief periods of gaze shifting (during which vision is poor) and longer periods of image stabilization (THB6 Figure 21-1, p. 525). Finally, animals with frontally directed eyes (again, like us) need to keep both foveae pointed at the same part of the world in order to make binocular depth perception possible; if this part of the system breaks down and the two images don't correspond, **diplopia** (double vision) results.

Two general kinds of movements are required to keep our eyes lined up this way. First, for objects at a constant distance from us we need to move both eyes the same amount in the same direction; these are called **conjugate** movements. Second, for objects at varying distances we need to either converge or diverge our eyes; these are appropriately called **vergence** movements. There are two distinctly different kinds of conjugate movements: fast ones called **saccades**, used to shift gaze or when something moves too fast to track, and slow ones that are used to stabilize images while we move or objects move.

Six Extraocular Muscles Move the Eye in the Orbit

We need to move each eye in various combinations of six directions. Four of them are obvious—medially (**adduction**), laterally (**abduction**), up (**elevation**), and down (**depression**). The two others are torsional movements, the kind you would make to keep an eye level as you tilt your head to one side or the other. **Intorsion** rotates the top of the eye closer to the nose and **extorsion** rotates it away. Movements in these six directions are accomplished by six small **extraocular muscles**, but the correspondence between movements and individual muscles is not always direct (Table 21-1).

The Medial and Lateral Recti Adduct and Abduct the Eye

Adduction and abduction are the most straightforward. They are accomplished by contraction of the **medial** and **lateral rectus**, respectively, which originate in the back of the orbit and insert on the medial and lateral sides of the eye.

The Superior and Inferior Recti and the Obliques Have More Complex Actions

The four remaining muscles—the **superior rectus**, **inferior rectus**, **superior oblique**, and **inferior oblique**—do not lie entirely in the same plane as one of the directions of eye movement, so their actions are more complex. For example, the eye (when looking at something far away) points straight ahead in the orbit, but the axis of the orbit itself—the direction in which the superior and inferior recti pull—points not only backward but also toward the nose (Fig. 21-1). The result is that contraction of the superior rectus mainly causes elevation, but also pulls the top of the eye toward the nose (i.e., intorsion and adduction). Similarly, the inferior rectus mainly causes

depression, but also causes extorsion and adduction. The superior and inferior obliques mainly cause intorsion and extorsion, respectively. However, because they insert behind the middle of the eye and pull partially anteriorly, they too cause movement in additional directions (see Table 21-1).

We ordinarily use all six muscles in most eye movements, exciting some motor neurons and inhibiting others, contracting some muscles and relaxing others. For example, abduction involves simultaneous contraction of not only the lateral rectus but also both obliques, as well as relaxation of the other three muscles. To keep things manageable, however, this chapter only considers vertical and horizontal movements and pretends they are mediated solely by contractions of the four rectus muscles.

There Are Fast and Slow Conjugate Eye Movements

There are two reasons for making conjugate eye movements: (1) to get an image onto the fovea and (2) to keep it there. Corresponding to this, there are two general categories of conjugate eye movements. Fast movements (saccades) get images onto the fovea and slower movements keep them there.

Table 21-1	Extraocular muscles, eye movements, and cranial nerves	
Movement	**Principal Muscle**	**Other Contributors**
Abduction	Lateral rectus (VI)	Inferior oblique (III) Superior oblique (IV)
Adduction	Medial rectus (III)	Inferior rectus (III) Superior rectus (III)
Depression	Inferior rectus (III)	Superior oblique (IV)
Elevation	Superior rectus (III)	Inferior oblique (III)
Extorsion	Inferior oblique (III)	Inferior rectus (III)
Intorsion	Superior oblique (III)	Superior rectus (III)

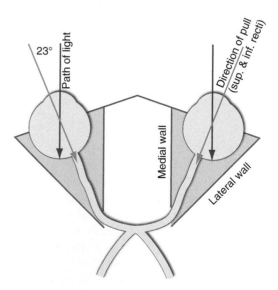

Figure 21-1 Visual and orbital axes. When looking straight ahead at something in the distance, the path of light goes through the middle of the pupil and lens and proceeds directly back to the fovea. The superior and inferior recti, however, are aligned with the middle of the orbit; because the lateral and medial orbital walls form an angle of about 45°, the direction in which these muscles pull is about 23° away from straight ahead.

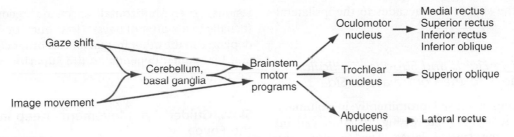

Figure 21-2 Overview of eye movement control systems. (This is just schematic and not meant to indicate, for example, that the basal ganglia project directly to brainstem motor programs for eye movements.)

Just as there are **motor programs** for things like walking that can be modulated by descending projections from places like motor cortex, there are groups of subcortical neurons specialized to generate the timing signals for fast and slow eye movements and pass them along to the oculomotor, trochlear, and abducens nuclei (Fig. 21-2). These timing centers receive inputs from those parts of the brain that can initiate eye movements and then send their outputs to the appropriate motor neurons; just as in the case of other movements, the cerebellum and basal ganglia play a role in planning and coordinating eye movements. Superimposed on this arrangement are projections from the **vestibular nuclei**, so that we can adjust eye position to compensate for head movements.

Fast, Ballistic Eye Movements Get Images onto the Fovea

> **Key Concept**
>
> Motor programs for saccades are located in the pons and midbrain.

Saccades are rapid conjugate movements (Fig. 21-3), in which our eyes can move as rapidly as 700°/second. We use saccades for voluntary eye movements, to look over at something we caught a glimpse of in the periphery, to catch up with something that's moving too fast to track, and as the fast phase of **nystagmus**. Moving your eyes like this is harder than it seems. It requires a very rapid burst (up to 1000 impulses/second) in the motor neurons to generate the velocity, and then a carefully calculated maintained firing rate to keep the eyes in their new position. Saccades are prepackaged movements, as though the brain calculates how far we need to move, sets up the timing, and then lets it fly. Once it starts, the saccade usually can't be changed, for example if the target moves again. One of the few ways a saccade

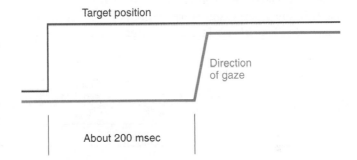

Figure 21-3 A saccade in response to abrupt movement of a target.

can be modified is through the vestibular nuclei. If you move your head during a saccade, the **vestibulo-ocular reflex** (VOR, see Fig. 14-11) automatically compensates for the movement.

The arrangement for vertical saccades is reasonably straightforward. The superior and inferior recti, both innervated by the oculomotor nerve, are the principal muscles. Corresponding to this, the timing machinery also lives in the rostral midbrain, both near the superior colliculi and posterior commissure and deeper in the midbrain, near the dorsomedial edge of the red nucleus. Things that press on the top of the midbrain, like pineal tumors, commonly cause a selective paralysis of upward gaze, and deeper damage can cause selective impairment of downward saccades.

For horizontal conjugate movements, things aren't quite that simple because we need to coordinate the lateral rectus of one eye with the medial rectus of the other eye. This is accomplished by having not only motor neurons in each abducens nucleus, but also interneurons that project through the contralateral MLF to the oculomotor nucleus (see Fig. 12-3). (These abducens interneurons are activated not just during saccades, but during all horizontal movements to the ipsilateral side.) The timing signals are generated in the **paramedian pontine reticular formation** (**PPRF**) near the abducens nucleus. The PPRF on one side of the pons sets up the signals for saccades to the ipsilateral side.

The Frontal Eye Fields and Superior Colliculus Trigger Saccades to the Contralateral Side

Because saccades are used prominently in voluntary eye movements, it is not surprising that they can be triggered from the frontal lobes. The specific area involved, called the **frontal eye field**, is just anterior to where the head is represented in motor cortex. A unilateral frontal lesion causes no problems with vertical saccades, so vertical eye movements are apparently represented bilaterally. In the case of horizontal saccades, each hemisphere triggers movements to the contralateral side (Fig. 21-4). However, after unilateral frontal

lesions, even horizontal saccades recover quickly (usually in a matter of days). How much of this recovery depends on the other frontal lobe or other cortical areas, and how much depends on the **superior colliculus**, is unclear.

Slow, Guided Eye Movements Keep Images on the Fovea

An image could move off the fovea if you moved or if the object moved. Corresponding to this, we have two different kinds of smooth, slower eye movements, one using vestibular feedback and the other using visual feedback. (The reason they are slower than saccades is that it takes time to produce and use this sensory feedback.)

The Vestibulo-ocular Reflex Compensates for Head Movement

You can keep an image on your fovea as you move around by using the VOR. If you don't want to keep an image on the fovea—for example, if you turn your head to look at something else—projections from the **flocculus** to the **vestibular nuclei** can turn it off.

Smooth Pursuit Movements Compensate for Target Movement

We use **pursuit** or **tracking** movements to track a moving object once its image is on or near the fovea. Pursuit movements can go at a maximum rate of only 50°/second or so. As a result, rapidly or irregularly moving objects require a combination of saccades and pursuit movements. Also, there's a latency of about 125 msec for pursuit movements when a target starts to move, so by the time we start to track something, its image has moved off the fovea; the CNS keeps track of all this and produces a catch-up saccade when required (Fig. 21-5).

Even though pursuit movements can get started faster than saccades (125 vs. 200 msec), they use what looks like a considerably more circuitous pathway. Signals from motion-sensitive areas of visual association cortex and from the frontal eye field reach a particular small group of pontine nuclei, and then in succession the flocculus, vestibular nuclei, and the abducens, trochlear, and oculomotor nuclei (Fig. 21-6). (This is probably because of an evolutionary relationship between pursuit movements and VOR suppression.) As in the case of saccades, vertical movements are triggered bilaterally. Oddly enough, each cerebral hemisphere is more involved in triggering horizontal pursuit movements to the ipsilateral side (probably a by-product of the evolutionary relationship to cerebellar circuitry).

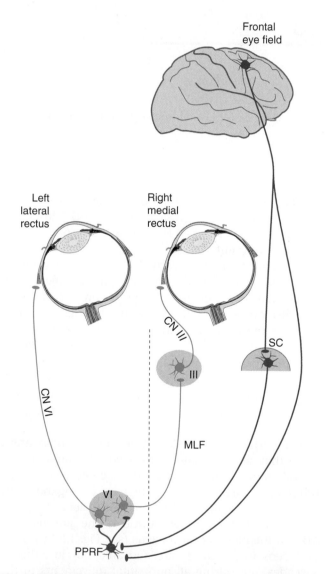

Figure 21-4 Circuitry for voluntary saccades to the left. *III*, Oculomotor nucleus; *MLF*, medial longitudinal fasciculus; *PPRF*, paramedian pontine reticular formation; *SC*, superior colliculus; *VI*, abducens nucleus.

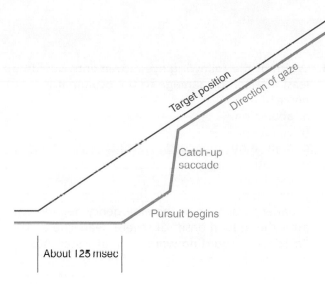
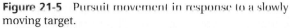

Target position

Direction of gaze

Catch-up saccade

Pursuit begins

About 125 msec

Figure 21-5   Pursuit movement in response to a slowly moving target.

Changes in Object Distance Require Vergence Movements

Vergence movements are part of the **near reflex** (see Fig. 17-9). The afferent limb of the reflex is the normal visual pathway from eyeball to occipital lobe. Visual association cortex of the occipital lobe then projects to the efferent machinery in the midbrain.

The Basal Ganglia and Cerebellum Participate in Eye Movement Control

Eye movements, like other movements, utilize the basal ganglia and cerebellum in their planning and coordination.

One of the parallel loops through the basal ganglia (see Fig. 19-4) passes through the frontal eye field and the **caudate nucleus** and **substantia nigra** (**reticular part**). This loop reaches not only the thalamus, but also the superior colliculus. Patients with basal ganglia disorders may have involuntary, small, or slow eye movements, much like the movements of other parts of their bodies.

The cerebellum gets involved in eye movements in several ways. As mentioned previously, the flocculus is

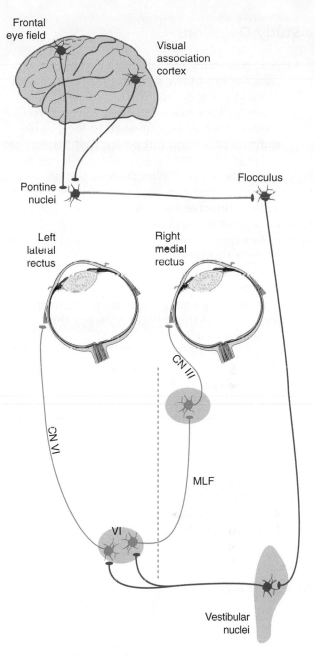
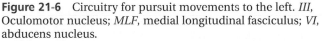

Figure 21-6   Circuitry for pursuit movements to the left. *III*, Oculomotor nucleus; *MLF*, medial longitudinal fasciculus; *VI*, abducens nucleus.

important for suppression of the VOR and for the production of smooth pursuit movements. In addition, part of the **vermis** (near where the head is represented) helps coordinate saccades; damage here can result in dysmetric saccades, much as cerebellar damage elsewhere can result in dysmetric limb movements.

Study Questions

1. A 39-year-old handball hustler comes to you complaining of the sudden onset of difficulty reading the sports pages, because he can't make his eyes move from left to right. You confirm that he cannot seem to look to his right on command but notice that his eyes can move to the right when you roll a handball across the floor. The most likely site of damage is his
   a. left abducens nucleus.
   b. right abducens nucleus.
   c. left frontal lobe.
   d. right frontal lobe.
   e. left MLF.
   f. right MLF.

2. The pathway and apparatus for the near reflex include all of the following *except* the
   a. oculomotor nucleus.
   b. visual cortex.
   c. MLF.
   d. pupillary sphincter.
   e. ciliary muscle.

3. The most important muscle for intorting the eye is the
   a. inferior oblique.
   b. inferior rectus.
   c. lateral rectus.
   d. medial rectus.
   e. superior oblique.
   f. superior rectus.

4. Which of the following eye movements would be least affected by damage to the oculomotor nerve?
   a. abduction.
   b. adduction.
   c. depression.
   d. elevation.
   e. extorsion.
   f. intorsion.

5. A patient was seen in the emergency department after the sudden onset of severe headache and "dizziness." Squirting warm or cool water into either ear caused nystagmus of normal amplitude and direction. However, when the patient tried to suppress the nystagmus by staring at a sign on the wall, she was unable to. The most likely site of damage was the
   a. basal ganglia.
   b. cerebellum.
   c. occipital lobes.

Cerebral Cortex

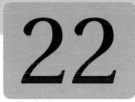

The cerebral cortex is ultimately the part of the CNS that makes us human. Other parts of the CNS like sensory pathways bring in raw data, the reticular activating system adjusts levels of excitability, but the cortex is where events are analyzed, plans are hatched, and responses are formulated. The cerebral cortex is a big sheet of repeated functional **modules**, with the operations of different arrays of modules corresponding to progressively more complex mental functions.

Most Cerebral Cortex Is Neocortex

Key Concepts

Pyramidal cells are the most numerous neocortical neurons.
Neocortex has six layers.

Most areas of cerebral cortex are **neocortex**, meaning that they have six more or less distinct **layers** (numbered **I** through **VI** from the surface down). About 80% of all cortical neurons are **pyramidal cells**, shaped as their name implies. They have a long **apical dendrite** ascending toward the cortical surface, a series of **basal dendrites**, and an axon emerging from the base of the cell body. Nearly all of the axons that leave the cerebral cortex are axons of pyramidal cells. The remaining 20% of cortical neurons is an assortment of **nonpyramidal cells**, most of them small and most of them inhibitory interneurons with axons that do not leave the cortex.

Layer I contains few cells and many synapses (just as the superficial layer of cerebellar cortex (see Chapter 20) is a place where mossy and climbing fibers synapse on the dendrites of Purkinje cells). Layer VI contains spindle-shaped modified pyramidal cells. The four middle layers of neocortex are alternating layers of mostly small cells and mostly large pyramidal cells (THB6 Figure 22-5, p. 545). Cortical areas that do not emit many long axons, such as primary sensory areas, are full of small pyramidal and nonpyramidal cells and are called **granular areas**. Cortical areas that emit many long axons, such as motor cortex, have many large pyramidal cells and are called **agranular areas**.

Different Neocortical Layers Have Distinctive Connections

The layering of neocortex is a mechanism for sorting its inputs and outputs. Afferents from other cortical areas (by far the majority), from the thalamus, and from modulatory nuclei in the brainstem and elsewhere distribute themselves in distinctive patterns among the various layers. Similarly, the pyramidal cells of any given layer have preferred targets; for example, layer V pyramids project to the striatum, brainstem, and spinal cord, and layer VI pyramids project to the thalamus.

The Corpus Callosum and Anterior Commissure Interconnect the Two Cerebral Hemispheres

One source of afferents from other cortical areas is the contralateral hemisphere. The **corpus callosum** is a bundle of several hundred million axons that interconnect the two cerebral hemispheres. Many of these fibers project from sites in the frontal, parietal, or occipital cortex on one side to the mirror-image sites on the other side. However, others interconnect areas that are functionally related to each other but not mirror images. Projections from the frontal lobes fill the **genu** and the anterior half of the **body** of the corpus callosum. The occipital lobes and parts of the temporal lobes project through the enlarged **splenium**, and the parietal lobes

through the posterior half of the body (THB6 Figure 22-28, p. 570).

The **anterior commissure** contains similar fibers that interconnect the rest of the temporal lobes, as well as other fibers that interconnect components of the olfactory system.

Association Bundles Interconnect Areas within Each Cerebral Hemisphere

The second general source of corticocortical afferents is other areas in the same hemisphere. Many of these travel in well-defined **association bundles**, but they are intermingled with other fiber bundles in the white matter of the cerebral hemisphere and not as obvious as the corpus callosum and anterior commissure. One functionally important association bundle is the **arcuate fasciculus**, which travels above the insula (THB6 Figure 22-9, p. 548); as described a little later, it interconnects two prominent language areas.

Neocortex Also Has a Columnar Organization

Despite the horizontal layering of neocortex, other data indicate that in a functional sense it is organized into **columns** on the order of 100 µm wide and oriented perpendicular to the cortical surface. Endings in one cortical area from either the thalamus or another cortical area are often organized into such columns, separated by other columns that do not receive such endings. Visual cortex is organized into columns of cells having similar response properties, with adjacent columns differing in some parameter (THB6 Figure 17-35, pp. 449 and 450). Likewise, somatosensory cortex is organized into columns of neurons that respond best to a particular kind of stimulus.

Neocortical Areas Are Specialized for Different Functions

> **Key Concept**
>
> Different neocortical areas have subtly different structures.

Although neocortex has the same basic structure everywhere in terms of percentages of pyramidal and nonpyramidal cells, layering, and columns, areas still differ from one another in terms of things like the sizes of cells and the thickness of layers. These differences turn out to be correlated with differences in function and connections, and so they have led to systematic maps of cortical areas. Several mapping systems have been devised, and some of the numbers in the map devised by Brodmann are in common use (THB6 Figure 22-10, p. 550). Important **Brodmann's numbers** are indicated in parentheses in the figures in this chapter.

There Are Sensory, Motor, Association, and Limbic Areas

Key Concepts

Primary somatosensory cortex is in the parietal lobe.
Primary visual cortex is in the occipital lobe.
Primary auditory cortex is in the temporal lobe.
There are primary vestibular, gustatory, and olfactory areas.
Most motor areas are in the frontal lobe.
Association areas mediate higher mental functions.
Parietal association cortex mediates spatial orientation.

Primary areas (Fig. 22-1) of cortex are those most directly linked to the rest of the world, either through inputs from thalamic sensory relay nuclei or through outputs to the brainstem and spinal cord. **Primary motor** cortex occupies part of the precentral gyrus, **primary somatosensory** cortex the postcentral gyrus, **primary auditory** cortex the transverse temporal gyri, and **primary visual** cortex the banks of the calcarine sulcus. These primary areas contain precise but distorted **somatotopic**, **tonotopic**, or **retinotopic** maps with large representations of

functionally important areas like the fingers, speech frequencies, and the fovea. There is also a **primary gustatory** area in the anterior insula and a **primary vestibular** area in the posterior insula, but relatively less is known about them. **Primary olfactory cortex** (see Chapter 13), in and near the anterior temporal lobe, is different in not being neocortical and not receiving its input from the thalamus.

Adjacent to each of the primary cortical areas are areas that are involved in the same function and that receive projections from the primary area (and usually from the appropriate thalamic relay nucleus as well). They have less precise somatotopic, tonotopic, and retinotopic maps than the primary areas, but their cells have more complex response properties. These are referred to as **unimodal** (i.e., single-function) **association areas** (Fig. 22-2). Corresponding to the great importance of vision for primates, there is a particularly large expanse of **visual association cortex**. Damage to unimodal areas can cause different kinds of sensory-specific **agnosia** (from a Greek word meaning "lack of knowledge"), in which someone is unable to recognize objects or some of their properties using a particular sensory modality even though basic sensation using that modality is normal; loss of the ability to recognize faces or colors (THB6 Box 17-2, p. 451) are two examples. Premotor cortex and the supplementary motor area are comparable unimodal areas adjacent to primary motor cortex.

The single-function association areas send converging outputs to two large expanses of more complex association cortex (Fig. 22-3). The first is a **parietal-occipital-temporal** region surrounded by sensory areas; it receives thalamic inputs from the **pulvinar** (which also projects to unimodal sensory association areas). The second is anterior to premotor cortex and is called **prefrontal**

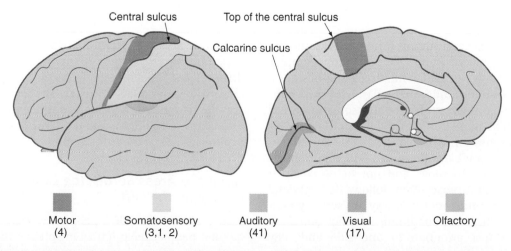

Figure 22-1   Primary sensory and motor areas, and Brodmann's numbers commonly associated with them. Not visible in this view are the gustatory and vestibular areas tucked away in the insula.

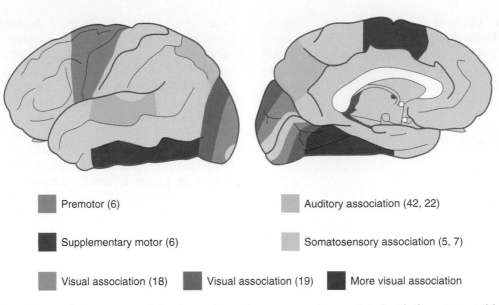

Figure 22-2 Unimodal association areas, and Brodmann's numbers commonly associated with them. Not visible in this view are gustatory and olfactory association areas in orbital cortex. There are additional vestibular areas, but it is not clear if one (or more) is comparable to other unimodal areas.

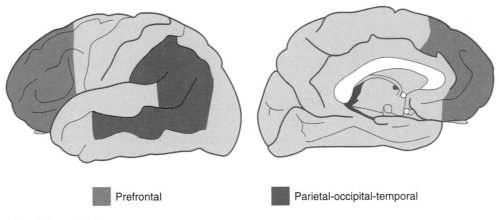

Figure 22-3 Multimodal association areas.

cortex; it receives thalamic inputs from the **dorsomedial nucleus**. Neurons in these areas have still more complex properties; they may respond to multiple kinds of stimuli and may only respond under particular behavioral conditions. Lesions in these **multimodal association areas** can cause deficits more complex than simple weakness or diminished sensation. **Apraxia** refers to a condition in which someone is unable to perform a skilled movement in spite of wanting to move and not being weak or uncoordinated, and most often follows left parietal damage. **Neglect syndromes** in a way are sensory analogs of apraxia. These are conditions in which someone is unable to direct attention to one side and may be totally unaware of one entire side of his or her body. Contralateral neglect most often follows damage to the right parietal or temporal lobe.

Limbic areas of cerebral cortex (Fig. 22-4), as described further in Chapter 23, operate in emotional and drive-related behavior by interconnecting the hypothalamus with other areas of cortex. The major limbic areas are the **cingulate** and **parahippocampal gyri**, with extensions onto the **insula**, the **temporal pole**, and the **orbital** surface of the frontal lobe.

Language Areas Border the Lateral Sulcus, Usually on the Left

Nearly all right-handed people, as well as most left-handed people, have left hemispheres that are **dominant** for the production and comprehension of language. Two areas in the left hemisphere are particularly important (Table 22-1). The posterior part of the left inferior

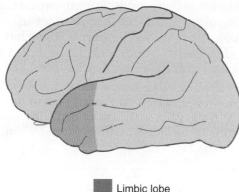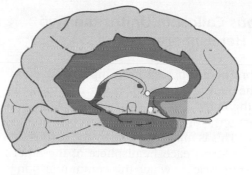

■ Limbic lobe   ■ Other limbic cortex

Figure 22-4 Limbic areas.

Table 22-1	Characteristics of major aphasia syndromes		
Aphasia	**Spontaneous Language**	**Comprehension**	**Repetition**
Broca's	Nonfluent, only essential words	Relatively OK	Poor
Wernicke's	Fluent, but defective content	Poor	Poor
Conduction	As in Wernicke's	Relatively OK	Poor
Global	Nonfluent	Poor	Poor

frontal gyrus, called **Broca's area**, is involved in the production of both written and spoken language. Damage affecting Broca's area and structures deep to it causes **nonfluent** (or **motor**, or **expressive**, or **Broca's**) **aphasia**, in which comprehension is relatively intact but language is produced only with difficulty. The posterior part of the left superior temporal gyrus, called **Wernicke's area**, is involved in the comprehension of both written and spoken language. Damage affecting Wernicke's area and adjoining cortex causes **fluent** (or **sensory**, or **receptive**, or **Wernicke's**) **aphasia**, in which language can be produced but its comprehension is relatively impaired. Affected individuals have difficulty comprehending even their own language, so it is produced fluidly but inaccurately; the result is incorrect words and meaningless phrases. Damage affecting the arcuate fasciculus (which interconnects Broca's area and Wernicke's area) and the overlying supramarginal gyrus causes **conduction aphasia**, in which an individual speaks and writes like a Wernicke's aphasic but comprehends language relatively well. Damage that encompasses both Broca's and Wernicke's areas causes **global aphasia**, in which both production and comprehension of language are impaired. Damage outside this **perisylvian language zone** (so called because it borders the Sylvian fissure, another name for the lateral sulcus) can cause other forms of nonfluent or fluent aphasia by removing important inputs to Broca's or Wernicke's area; because connections between auditory cortex and these language areas are still intact, however, such patients are still able to repeat spoken words.

The Right and Left Cerebral Hemispheres Are Specialized for Different Functions

The left hemisphere of most people is dominant not only for language, but also for mathematical ability, planning skilled movements, and logical, sequential analysis. The right hemisphere, in contrast, is better with spatial and musical patterns and better at solving problems in a more intuitive fashion. The right hemisphere equivalents of Broca's and Wernicke's areas are important for the production and recognition of the rhythmic and musical aspects (**prosody**) of language that convey much of its emotional meaning.

Prefrontal Cortex Mediates Working Memory and Decision Making

Prefrontal cortex receives inputs from sensory and motor association areas, as well as limbic areas. It uses these inputs to concentrate on things and keep them in **working memory**, and also to play a major role in various aspects of personality like initiative, social interaction, insight, and foresight. Dorsal and lateral prefrontal areas are more important for working memory, attention, and logical aspects of problem solving. Orbital and medial areas have extensive limbic connections and are more important for emotional aspects of plans and decisions. Bilateral prefrontal damage may cause little change in basic intelligence but can cause emotional lability or flattening, difficulty maintaining attention, diminished drive and curiosity, and decreased creativity. Unilateral prefrontal damage can cause similar but less pronounced changes.

The Corpus Callosum Unites the Two Cerebral Hemispheres

Our two cerebral hemispheres receive inputs from opposite sides of the body or the outside world, control opposite sides of the body, and are specialized for different cognitive functions, yet we experience a single, unified consciousness. This is made possible by the corpus callosum, which informs each hemisphere of the other's activities. The rare cases in which this communication is disrupted result in peculiar abnormalities reflecting independent operation of the two hemispheres. For example, such a patient might be unable to describe verbally any stimuli reaching the right hemisphere because that hemisphere would be unable to convey the relevant information to language areas in the left hemisphere.

Disconnection Syndromes Can Result from White Matter Damage

Normal function of an area of cerebral cortex depends not only on the cortex itself, but also on its input and output connections. Hence, disconnection of cortical areas from one another can produce functional deficits similar to those resulting from cortical damage. Sectioning of the corpus callosum provides an extreme example of a **disconnection syndrome**. There have been cases in which motor cortex was disconnected from language areas, with the result that an individual was unable to make movements upon request and so appeared to be apraxic. Similarly, disconnection of visual cortex from language areas can render someone unable to read in spite of having otherwise normal vision and language comprehension.

Consciousness and Sleep Are Active Processes

Consciousness—the waking state of self-awareness—is a result of interactions between the cerebral cortex and other parts of the nervous system. The **content** of consciousness is a reflection of moment-to-moment interactions between different cortical areas; the **level** of consciousness is regulated by diffuse modulatory projections to the thalamus and cortex (Fig. 22-5). Some of these, as mentioned in Chapter 11, are projections from the **ascending reticular activating system** (**ARAS**) in the brainstem; others arise in the hypothalamus and basal

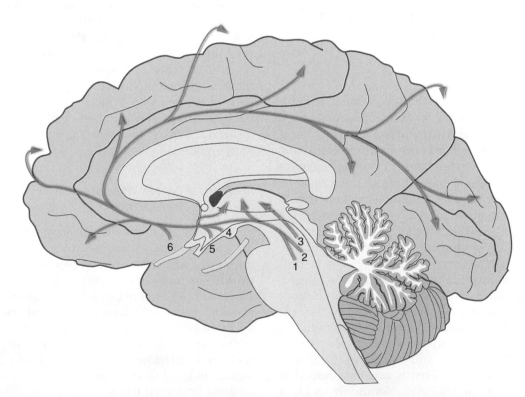

Figure 22-5 Major sources of diffuse modulatory projections to the thalamus and cortex that affect the level of consciousness. *1*, Raphe nuclei (serotonin); *2*, locus ceruleus (norepinephrine); *3*, midbrain reticular formation (acetylcholine); *4*, posterior hypothalamus, near the mammillary bodies (histamine); *5*, lateral hypothalamus, near the fornix (orexin); *6*, basal nucleus (acetylcholine). All of these groups of neurons project to both the thalamus and the cortex, except for 3 (to the thalamus) and 6 (to the cortex).

forebrain. Major components include chemically coded neurons in the rostral pons and midbrain (e.g., noradrenergic, serotonergic), hypothalamic neurons that use **histamine** or **orexin** (a neuropeptide) as a neurotransmitter, and cholinergic neurons in the basal nucleus and the midbrain reticular formation. Collectively, this network of modulatory neurons regulates the level of excitability of the cortex and helps switch thalamic neurons back and forth between tonic and bursting modes.

Loss of consciousness is always the result of bilaterally diminished activity in large areas of cerebral cortex, large parts of the diffuse modulatory network, or the diencephalon. **Coma** can result from metabolic or vascular events that inactivate or damage large areas of both cerebral hemispheres, or from bilateral damage to the diencephalon or ARAS, but not from unilateral damage. Sleep is a temporary loss of consciousness that results from active processes that "turn off" some of the consciousness-generating interactions bilaterally.

There Are Two Forms of Sleep

> ### Key Concept
>
> Control circuits for REM sleep are located in the brainstem.

During wakefulness the electroencephalogram (EEG) typically is either a small, desynchronized signal (during attentiveness) or contains small, synchronized waves in an 8 to 13 Hz alpha rhythm (during relaxation). As we fall asleep, the waking desynchronized EEG gives way in stages to a more and more synchronized, slow-wave signal (delta waves, <4 Hz). These stages of **non-REM sleep**, culminating in **slow-wave sleep**, are interrupted periodically by intervals of **REM sleep**, in which there is a desynchronized EEG like that of wakefulness, accompanied by detailed dreams and bursts of rapid eye movements (Table 22-2).

Table 22-2	Non-REM and REM sleep	
	Non-REM Sleep	**REM Sleep**
EEG	Progressively bigger, slower, more synchronized	Small, fast, desynchronized
Muscle tone	Somewhat reduced	Almost abolished
Arousal threshold	High	Higher
Mental activity	Vague dreams	Detailed, complex dreams
ANS activity	Increased parasympathetic; slow, regular pulse and respiration	Increased sympathetic; irregular pulse and respiration

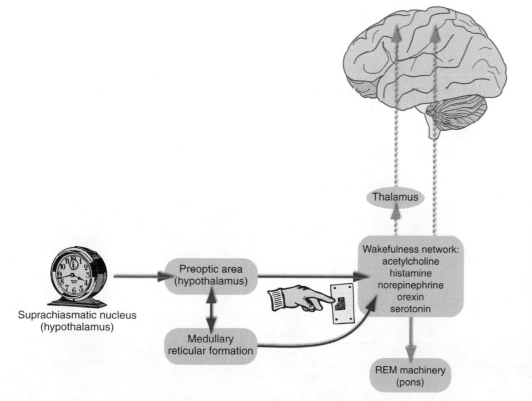

Figure 22-6　Sleep circuitry. With a periodicity orchestrated by the suprachiasmatic nucleus, the preoptic area and medullary reticular formation turn off the wakefulness-promoting network. While this network is off, REM machinery in the pons gets turned on with its own period of about 90 minutes.

Both Brainstem and Forebrain Mechanisms Regulate Sleep-Wake Transitions

Coordinated activity of the most anterior part of the hypothalamus (the preoptic area; see Chapter 23) and the reticular formation of the caudal brainstem periodically inhibits the wakefulness-promoting network shown in Fig. 22-5, and we fall asleep (Fig. 22-6). Sleep is something we do regularly, with a period of about 24 hours. The clock that controls the sleep-wakefulness cycle is in the **suprachiasmatic nucleus** of the hypothalamus (see Chapter 23); its output gets in step with the day-night cycle through retinal inputs to the suprachiasmatic nucleus and is then passed along to the preoptic area. Reduced activity in the wakefulness-promoting network in turn reduces cortical activity, and slow-wave sleep is the result. REM sleep, in contrast, depends on neural machinery located in the pons that turns on and off about every 90 minutes during periods of slow-wave sleep (THB6 Figure 22-35, p. 576).

Study Questions

1. The principal output neurons of the cerebral cortex are
   a. stellate cells.
   b. granule cells.
   c. Purkinje cells.
   d. pyramidal cells.
2. Most of the fibers in the anterior commissure interconnect the
   a. frontal lobes.
   b. parietal lobes.
   c. occipital lobes.
   d. temporal lobes.

11. REM sleep and slow-wave sleep are similar in that
    a. relative to wakefulness, the EEG in both states is of smaller amplitude.
    b. both are characterized by detailed visual dreams.
    c. muscle tone is almost abolished.
    d. the basic neural machinery for both is in the thalamus.
    e. none of the above.

Answer questions 3 through 10 using the following diagram. Each letter may be used once, more than once, or not at all.

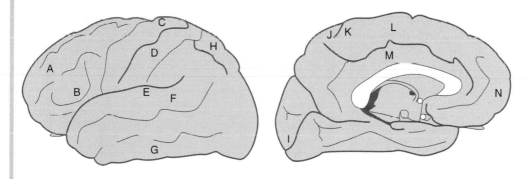

3. Area 17.
4. Agranular cortex.
5. Somatosensory association cortex.
6. Limbic cortex.
7. Supplementary motor area.
8. Area 6.
9. Damage here would cause problems comprehending language.
10. In the right hemisphere, damage here might cause speech to be flat and monotonic.

Drives and Emotions: The Hypothalamus and Limbic System

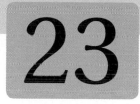

There is a whole sphere of mental activity that goes beyond simple perception of stimuli and logical formulation of responses. We have drives and urges, and most of our experiences are emotionally colored. This emotional coloring and its relationship with basic drives is the province of the **limbic system**. The **hypothalamus** regulates autonomic function and drive-related behavior, and limbic structures serve as bridges between the hypothalamus and neocortex.

The Hypothalamus Coordinates Drive-Related Behaviors

The hypothalamus is a nodal point in the neural circuits underlying drive-related behaviors (Fig. 23-1). It's got interconnections with visceral parts of the nervous system, through which it is informed of and controls things like blood glucose, blood pressure, and body temperature. It's

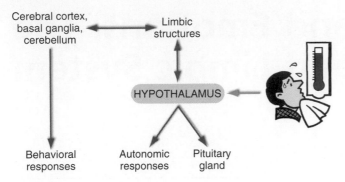

Figure 23-1 Overview of limbic and hypothalamic roles in responses to environmental changes.

also got interconnections with limbic structures, through which you become aware of homeostatic needs ("I'm hungry"). Finally, the hypothalamus has not just neural outputs but also ways to control the **pituitary gland**.

The Hypothalamus Can Be Subdivided in Both Longitudinal and Medial-Lateral Directions

Parts of the hypothalamus are exposed at the base of the brain, surrounded by the circle of Willis. The **mammillary bodies** form the most posterior part of the hypothalamus and lie adjacent to the cerebral peduncles. Between the mammillary bodies and the optic chiasm and tract is a small swelling called the **tuber cinereum**. The **median eminence** arises from the tuber cinereum and narrows into the **infundibulum**, to which the pituitary gland is attached. These landmarks on the base of the brain are used to divide the hypothalamus longitudinally (Fig. 23-2) into an **anterior region** (above the

optic chiasm, extending anteriorly to the lamina terminalis), a **tuberal region** (above and including the tuber cinereum), and a **posterior region** (above and including the mammillary bodies).

The hypothalamus also gets divided up in a medial to lateral direction. The periaqueductal gray of the midbrain continues into the thin **periventricular zone** in the wall of the third ventricle. The **fornix** runs right through the longitudinal zones on its way to the mammillary body and is used as a landmark to divide the rest of the hypothalamus on each side into **medial** and **lateral zones**.

Hypothalamic Inputs Arise in Widespread Neural Sites

Key Concepts

Most inputs from the forebrain arise in limbic structures.

Inputs from the brainstem and spinal cord traverse the medial forebrain bundle and dorsal longitudinal fasciculus.

The hypothalamus contains intrinsic sensory neurons.

The hypothalamus receives lots of inputs (Fig. 23-3), but most of them are from two general categories: those from nuclei in the brainstem and spinal cord conveying information about the state of your body, and those from limbic structures like the **amygdala**, **hippocampus**, and **septal nuclei**. Inputs about the state of the body ("It's getting warm in here," or "Blood glucose is getting low") arrive from places like the **nucleus of the solitary tract** by way of the **dorsal longitudinal fasciculus**, which travels through the periaqueductal gray into the periventricular zone; through the **medial forebrain bundle**, which travels through the reticular formation into the

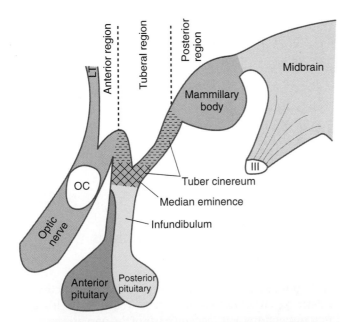

Figure 23-2 Longitudinal subdivisions of the hypothalamus, and the two lobes of the pituitary gland. *III*, Oculomotor nerve; *LT*, lamina terminalis (the membrane at the anterior end of the third ventricle); *OC*, optic chiasm.

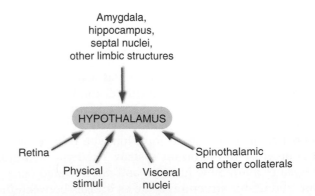

Figure 23-3 Inputs to the hypothalamus.

lateral hypothalamus; and as branches from tracts like the spinothalamic tract. Limbic inputs arrive from the amygdala, from the hippocampus (through the fornix), and from the septal nuclei and other sites (through the medial forebrain bundle); collectively they keep the hypothalamus updated on other aspects of the environment ("Not a good place to take off my shirt").

Inputs also reach the hypothalamus from the retina and in the form of direct physical stimuli. Axons of some retinal ganglion cells terminate in the small **suprachiasmatic nucleus** on each side of the anterior hypothalamus. The suprachiasmatic nucleus is the "master clock" for most **circadian rhythms**, and information from the retina helps get these rhythms synchronized with the 24-hour day (THB6 Figure 23-5, p. 585). Finally, some hypothalamic neurons are sensory receptors themselves, directly responsive to temperature, blood osmolality, or the concentration of some chemicals in blood passing through the hypothalamus.

Hypothalamic Outputs Largely Reciprocate Inputs

Hypothalamic connections with visceral nuclei and limbic structures are largely reciprocal (Fig. 23-4). Projections through the dorsal longitudinal fasciculus and the medial forebrain bundle reach sites like the nucleus of the solitary tract, the **dorsal motor nucleus of the vagus**, and the **intermediolateral cell column** of the spinal cord ("Better start sweating"). Projections through the medial forebrain bundle and other routes reach the amygdala, septal nuclei, and other limbic structures ("Maybe I can find the thermostat"). (Hypothalamic output reaches the hippocampus through a more circuitous route utilizing the thalamus, as described in Chapter 24.) In addition, diffuse modulatory projections to the thalamus and cerebral cortex play a key role in sleep-wake cycles (see Figs. 22-5 and 22-6).

The Hypothalamus Controls Both Lobes of the Pituitary Gland

The final, and major, hypothalamic outputs control the pituitary gland (**hypophysis**) through two separate

mechanisms (Fig. 23-5). (1) Hypothalamic neurons in the **supraoptic** and **paraventricular** nuclei are the source of **antidiuretic hormone** (**vasopressin**) and **oxytocin**. They transport these hormones down their axons to the **posterior lobe** of the pituitary (most of the **neurohypophysis**), where they are released into the circulation. (2) Hypothalamic neurons in and near the tuber cinereum produce small peptides that serve as **releasing** and **inhibiting factors** for the **anterior lobe** of the pituitary (most of the **adenohypophysis**). They transport these factors down their axons and release them into capillaries in the median eminence. These capillaries then converge into pituitary **portal vessels** that travel down the infundibular stalk to a second capillary bed in the anterior pituitary. The releasing and inhibiting factors leave the second capillary bed and control the production of anterior pituitary hormones.

Perforating Branches from the Circle of Willis Supply the Hypothalamus

The infundibular stalk sits right in the middle of the circle of Willis (THB6 Figure 6-3, p. 126), suggesting where the blood supply of the hypothalamus comes from—small perforating or ganglionic branches all around the circle.

The Hypothalamus Collaborates with a Network of Brainstem and Spinal Cord Neurons

The connections of the hypothalamus position it to control the whole gamut of homeostatic mechanisms and drive-related behaviors—temperature regulation, feeding and drinking, cardiovascular function, sexual

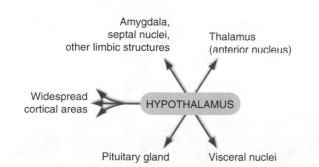

Figure 23-4   Outputs from the hypothalamus.

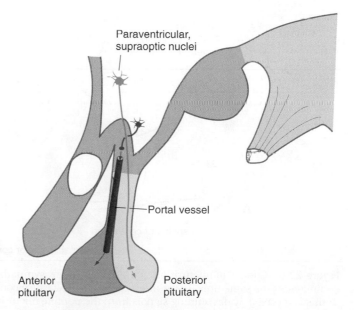

Figure 23-5   Hypothalamic control of the pituitary gland.

behavior, hormonal regulation, aggression, and on and on. Although some of these activities mainly involve autonomic adjustments (e.g., cardiovascular reflexes), skeletal muscle plays a major role in others (e.g., breathing). Normal control of **micturition (urination)** provides a nice example of coordination among visceral afferents, conscious awareness, smooth muscle, skeletal muscle, and voluntary control.

Normal Micturition Involves a Central Pattern Generator in the Pons

The bladder is a container that spends most of its time storing urine; it can do this because the pressure inside the bladder is usually low—the smooth muscle in its wall (the **detrusor**) is relaxed, and the **internal** (smooth muscle) and **external** (skeletal muscle) **sphincters** in its neck are contracted. This **storage mode** is maintained by sympathetic inputs and by tonic firing of motor neurons to the external sphincter (Fig. 23-6A). Periodically the sphincters relax, the detrusor contracts, and urine is eliminated. Infants do this automatically, using spinal cord reflex circuitry that is suppressed later in life. For adults, entering this **elimination mode** is more complicated because decisions need to be made about appropriate times and places to urinate. The **periaqueductal gray** sums up inputs from the spinal cord (tension in the bladder wall), the hypothalamus, and cerebral cortex, then passes the decision along to the

pontine micturition center, which executes it (Fig. 23-6B).

Damage at various levels of the CNS causes an array of deficits in bladder control analogous to those affecting skeletal muscle. Lesions of the sacral spinal cord or cauda equina are much like lower motor neuron damage: The detrusor is unable to contract, so the bladder expands under relatively low pressure. Eventually enough pressure builds up for some urine to be expelled, but the bladder never empties. Damage between the midthoracic spinal cord and the pontine micturition center, in contrast, is like an upper motor neuron lesion. Spinal cord reflexes reemerge and become hyperactive, so the bladder tries to empty itself even when the volume is low. The external sphincter never gets a signal from the pontine micturition center telling it to relax, however, so the detrusor has to contract really hard to produce enough pressure to overcome it. Damage above the pons leaves all this circuitry intact but can remove some inputs to the pontine micturition center, causing a variety of problems like increased urgency or diminished social awareness.

The Hypothalamus and Associated Central Pattern Generators Keep Physiological Variables within Narrow Limits

In a similar way, the hypothalamus monitors a host of other physiological variables and is involved in initiating

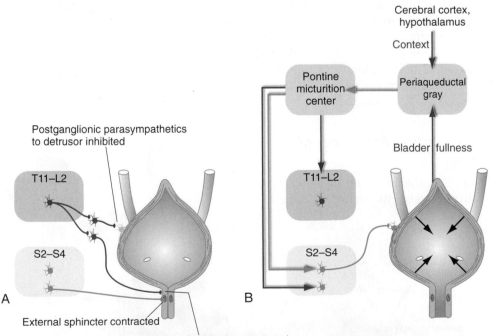

Figure 23-6 Control of micturition. **A,** In storage mode, sympathetic innervation relaxes the detrusor and contracts the internal sphincter. At the same time, lower motor neurons in S2 cause contraction of the external sphincter. **B,** In elimination mode, all of this is reversed by descending signals from the pontine micturition center.

the right mix of autonomic, hormonal, and behavioral responses to changes in these variables—secreting more antidiuretic hormone in response to increased plasma osmolality, for example, while at the same time contributing to a feeling of thirst through interactions with the limbic system.

Limbic Structures Are Interposed between the Hypothalamus and Neocortex

We perceive multiple attributes of things—not only their physical attributes, but also whether they are attractive, frightening, and so on. Integration of these multiple attributes occurs in the multimodal association areas of the cerebral cortex (see Fig. 22-3), using multiple inputs. Information about physical attributes comes from the unimodal association areas, whereas information about their drive-related attributes comes from limbic structures. Drive-related attributes of objects or situations also have implications for autonomic and behavioral responses, and these are mediated by the same limbic structures in conjunction with the hypothalamus and the adjacent septal area. Hence, the general notion of the limbic system is that limbic structures serve as a sort of bridge between neocortex and behavior when drives and emotions are involved (see Fig. 23-1).

The Hippocampus and Amygdala Are the Central Components of the Two Major Limbic Subsystems

The limbic system includes both cortical areas and noncortical structures and is divided into two subsystems, one centered on the **hippocampus** and the other on the **amygdala**. Each uses different areas of cerebral cortex as part of the bridge to multimodal association areas. The hippocampal subsystem is primarily involved in learning and memory, as described in Chapter 24.

The Amygdala Is Centrally Involved in Emotional Responses

> **Key Concepts**
>
> The amygdala receives a wide variety of sensory inputs.
> The amygdala projects to the cerebral cortex and hypothalamus.

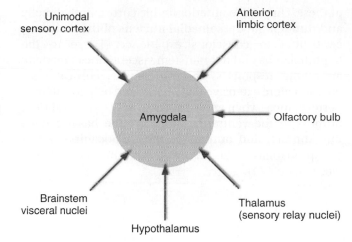

Figure 23-7 Inputs to the amygdala.

The amygdala, a collection of nuclei located in the temporal lobe at the anterior end of the hippocampus, is a key link between experiences and emotional reactions to them. It receives a great deal of sensory information of all sorts, from the brainstem, thalamus, hypothalamus, olfactory bulb, and unimodal association areas (Fig. 23-7). It also receives inputs from anterior parts of the limbic lobe and nearby areas, including **orbital** and **anterior temporal** cortex and the **insula**. Connections with the hypothalamus travel through both the **stria terminalis** and a more diffuse pathway that passes underneath the lenticular nucleus. The stria terminalis, like the fornix, curves around with the lateral ventricle, but in this case travels just medial to the caudate nucleus; for much of its course it lies in the groove between the caudate nucleus and the thalamus.

Emotional experiences are accompanied by conscious awareness of the emotion, autonomic reactions, and heightened awareness of ongoing events, and outputs from the amygdala (Fig. 23-8) help mediate all

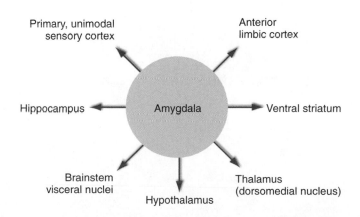

Figure 23-8 Outputs from the amygdala.

of these. Outputs to anterior limbic cortex, both directly and through the **dorsomedial nucleus** of the thalamus, contribute to conscious experience. Those to the hypothalamus and to brainstem visceral nuclei mediate autonomic responses. Those to sensory cortical areas are even more extensive than inputs and help to enhance performance when the pressure is on. In addition, outputs to the ventral striatum get the basal ganglia into the act, and outputs to the hippocampus affect the probability that an event will be remembered (see Chapter 24).

The Amygdala Is Involved in Emotion-Related Aspects of Learning

The amygdala uses its interconnections with limbic and sensory cortex and the hypothalamus both to form and to express associations between objects and the reactions they provoke. That is, while the hippocampus is important for remembering that an event occurred (see Chapter 24), the amygdala is important not only for remembering whether the event was "good" or "bad," but also for triggering appropriate responses ("gut feelings") the next time a similar event occurs.

Study Questions

1. The landmark that separates the lateral and medial zones of the hypothalamus is the
   a. anterior commissure.
   b. dorsal longitudinal fasciculus.
   c. fornix.
   d. medial forebrain bundle.
   e. stria terminalis.

2. The mammillary bodies are part of the _____ region of the hypothalamus.
   a. anterior
   b. tuberal
   c. posterior
   d. lateral

3. The timekeeping neurons that control most circadian rhythms are located in the
   a. amygdala.
   b. hippocampus.
   c. paraventricular nucleus.
   d. suprachiasmatic nucleus.
   e. supraoptic nucleus.

4. Production of anterior pituitary hormones is controlled by
   a. direct neural input from the supraoptic and paraventricular nuclei.
   b. direct neural input from neurons in the tuber cinereum.
   c. hormones secreted by the supraoptic and paraventricular nuclei and released into hypothalamic blood vessels.
   d. releasing and inhibiting factors secreted into the pituitary portal circulation by hypothalamic neurons.

5. The stria terminalis interconnects the _____ and the _____.
   a. amygdala, hippocampus
   b. amygdala, hypothalamus
   c. cingulate gyrus, parahippocampal gyrus
   d. nucleus of the solitary tract, hypothalamus

6. Most or all neurons that use histamine as a neurotransmitter are located in the
   a. amygdala.
   b. brainstem.
   c. hippocampus.
   d. hypothalamus.
   e. septal nuclei.

7. During the period in which a normal bladder is filling, the firing rates of sacral parasympathetic neurons, lumbar sympathetic neurons, and neurons in the pontine micturition center are, respectively,
   a. high, high, high.
   b. high, high, low.
   c. high, low, high.
   d. high, low, low.
   e. low, low, low.
   f. low, low, high.
   g. low, high, low.
   h. low, high, high.

8. The amygdala receives substantial inputs from
   a. built in temperature-sensitive neurons.
   b. the dorsal motor nucleus of the vagus.
   c. primary visual cortex.
   d. the ventral striatum.
   e. visual association cortex.

9. Efferents from the amygdala to the thalamus mostly terminate in the _____ nucleus.
   a. anterior
   b. dorsomedial
   c. lateral geniculate
   d. pulvinar
   e. ventral lateral

10. A 39-year-old handball hustler reported that every time he looked at a court where he had lost a match in the finals of a tournament the previous year, his blood pressure went up. The most important neural link underlying this reaction was a projection from the _____ to the _____.
    a. amygdala, hippocampus
    b. amygdala, hypothalamus
    c. amygdala, thalamus
    d. hippocampus, amygdala
    e. hypothalamus, amygdala
    f. thalamus, hypothalamus

Formation, Modification, and Repair of Neuronal Connections

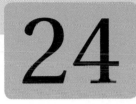

The nervous system is a lot less able to repair itself after damage than some other organs are, but that doesn't mean it can't change. There's extensive adjustment of connections during development, but even in adult brains synapses all over the nervous system modify their strength over time scales ranging from seconds to years. Some of these modifications are the basis of normal learning and memory.

There is hope that enhancing adult **plasticity**, or reactivating developmental plasticity, will make much greater levels of neurological repair possible in the near future.

Both Neurons and Connections Are Produced in Excess during Development

Similar developmental processes are at work in the formation of animals with bodies as different as snakes, star-nosed moles, and humans, and each needs a nervous system matched to its body. For example, humans need more motor neurons in the spinal cord segments that supply limbs (THB6 Figure 10-8, p. 236), but snakes do not. This could be done by starting out with a baseline number of neurons in each cord segment and adding more where needed, but in fact an exactly opposite approach is taken. Spinal cord segments, and all other parts of the CNS, start out with more neurons than they will ever need and the extras die during development. Similarly, each neuron starts out with more processes than it will ever need, and the extras get pruned away during development.

Collectively, these processes of developmental plasticity result in nervous systems that are matched to the bodies and environments they live in. The downside of this strategy is that environmental abnormalities during development can lead to permanently miswired nervous systems.

Neurotrophic Factors Ensure That Adequate Numbers of Neurons Survive

A critical factor that determines whether a given neuron survives or dies during development is its success in accumulating **neurotrophic factors** of specific kinds, different kinds for different neuronal types (Fig. 24-1). Neurotrophic factors are produced in limited amounts by target tissues (e.g., muscle, glands, other neurons), gobbled up by presynaptic endings, and transported back to the cell body. There they act to prevent **apoptosis** (programmed cell death) and to promote growth. Going back to the spinal cord example, more dorsal root ganglion cells and motor neurons survive at levels where there's a lot of target tissue in the periphery (e.g., lower cervical) than at levels where there's less (e.g., midthoracic). But this isn't restricted to the spinal cord—

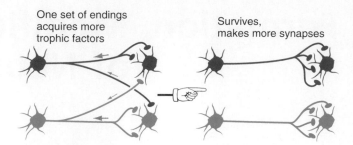

Figure 24-2 Competition for trophic factors leading to survival and proliferation of axonal branches during development.

throughout the nervous system, something like half of all the neurons produced during development die before birth.

Axonal Branches Are Pruned to Match Functional Requirements

Long after neurons finish competing with each other for survival, they continue to compete for neurotrophic factors in an effort to preserve their connections (Fig. 24-2).

The best-known example is the innervation of skeletal muscle by lower motor neurons. Early on, individual muscle fibers receive inputs from multiple motor neurons. By about the time of birth, all but one input has been pruned away and the sole survivor develops into a single elaborate neuromuscular junction (THB6 Figure 8-11, p. 184). Similar pruning goes on throughout the nervous system; depending on the area involved, this is a process that may continue well after birth.

Pruning of Neuronal Connections Occurs during Critical Periods

Neuronal connections are pruned and refined during limited time windows called **critical periods**. These are periods during which patterns of connections are fine-tuned, largely completing the process of matching the nervous system to the body and environment; once they end, further change is much more difficult. The downside here is that the decreased plasticity makes it difficult to repair things after damage to adult nervous systems.

The timing of critical periods is roughly correlated with the complexity of neural functions. This makes sense because, for example, multimodal cortical areas can't finish refining their connections until after unimodal areas are done. Some patterns of connections (e.g., innervation of skeletal muscle) are finalized at birth or earlier. Others (e.g., subtleties of language) continue for another decade or longer (THB6 Figure 24-9, p. 615).

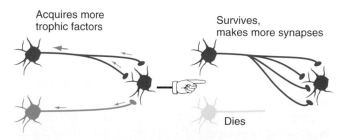

Figure 24-1 Competition for trophic factors and its effects on neuronal survival during development.

This has important clinical implications: abnormalities in eyes, ears, and social situations early in life need to be avoided or corrected in order to prevent permanent deficits.

Synaptic Connections Are Adjusted throughout Life

Critical periods can't be the end of the story, though, because changes in synaptic strength continue throughout life. Some of the changes last no more than a few minutes, but others last hours to years, long enough to play key roles in things like learning and memory. Changes in presynaptic or postsynaptic Ca^{2+} concentration play an important part in many, but not all, of these changes.

There Are Short-Term and Long-Term Adjustments of Synaptic Strength

> **Key Concept**
>
> Cortical maps are adjusted throughout life.

Some of the short-term changes in synaptic strength follow naturally from normal synaptic function (Fig. 24-3). A little extra Ca^{2+} hanging around in a presynaptic terminal after transmitter release, for example, can result in **potentiation** of transmitter release in response to the next action potential. High-frequency stimulation of a presynaptic ending can cause depletion of synaptic ves-

icles, resulting in **depression** of subsequent release for a little while. Fast-acting retrograde messengers, such as nitric oxide, can also cause short-term changes.

Longer-term changes can involve almost any conceivable part of presynaptic or postsynaptic elements (THB6 Figure 24-10, p. 616). One prominent example is the insertion or removal of postsynaptic transmitter receptors, resulting in **long-term potentiation** (**LTP**) or **long-term depression** (**LTD**). This can be triggered by postsynaptic Ca^{2+} entry through **NMDA receptors** (Fig. 24-4). NMDA receptors (named for *N*-methyl-D-aspartate, which binds to them) are glutamate receptors with some special properties. First, they only open when they bind glutamate *and* the membrane is already depolarized, making them great detectors of simultaneous activity at multiple synapses—something that could be a building block for memory formation. Second, they are

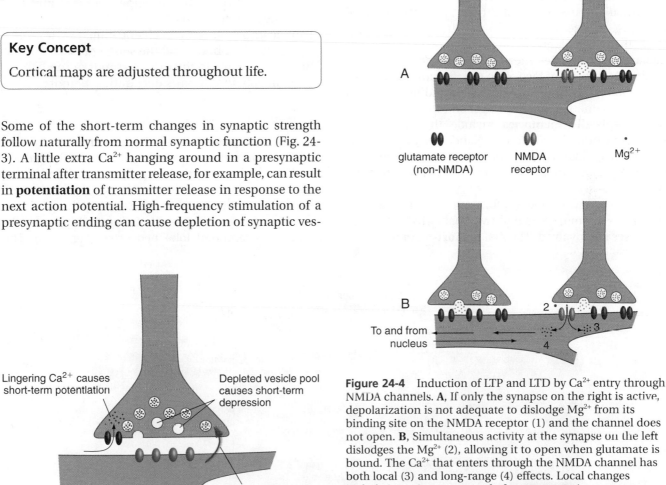

Figure 24-3 A few mechanisms of short-term changes in synaptic strength.

Lingering Ca^{2+} causes short-term potentiation

Depleted vesicle pool causes short-term depression

Fast-acting retrograde signals

glutamate receptor (non-NMDA)

NMDA receptor

Mg^{2+}

To and from nucleus

Figure 24-4 Induction of LTP and LTD by Ca^{2+} entry through NMDA channels. **A**, If only the synapse on the right is active, depolarization is not adequate to dislodge Mg^{2+} from its binding site on the NMDA receptor (1) and the channel does not open. **B**, Simultaneous activity at the synapse on the left dislodges the Mg^{2+} (2), allowing it to open when glutamate is bound. The Ca^{2+} that enters through the NMDA channel has both local (3) and long-range (4) effects. Local changes include insertion or removal of neurotransmitter receptors (causing LTP or LTD, respectively). Long-range effects include interactions with the nucleus, resulting in changes in the synthesis of neurotransmitter receptors and other synaptic molecules.

less selective than other ion channels and let Ca^{2+} through (in addition to Na^+ and K^+). Small amounts of Ca^{2+} entry cause LTD, and larger amounts cause LTP. Subsequent Ca^{2+}-initiated communication with the nucleus can make these changes very long lasting.

Modifications of synaptic strength play a big role in lifelong adjustments of cortical maps. These maps were traditionally considered to be static, but in fact the concentrated use of some body part or input (e.g., intense practice with a musical instrument) causes the corresponding part of the map to expand. Conversely, restricted use (e.g., having an arm in a cast) causes the representation to shrink. The changes in maps begin to happen within hours, much too quickly to involve growth of new connections.

Multiple Memory Systems Depend on Adjustments of Synaptic Strength

Most of us associate memory with things like learning lists of items before taking a test or writing a book, but there are actually multiple types of memory, each related to particular parts of the CNS (Fig. 24-5). Memories of facts (e.g., whose picture is on a dollar bill) and events (e.g., the particulars of the last handball game) are **declarative memories**, meaning you can *declare* them to be true. Memories of facts, also called **semantic memories**, span a range of categories, including historical facts, mathematical relationships, and the meanings of words; **episodic memories** include the specifics of events, including their timing. **Nondeclarative memories**, such as skills, patterns of behavior, and emotional reactions, are learned over time but show up more subconsciously.

A simple view of how we form memories, especially declarative memories, is that two qualitatively different processes are involved. The first is **short-term memory**, a process that depends on directed attention and continuous neuronal activity. Disruption of this process, for example by temporary loss of consciousness, causes loss of all items in short-term memory. Short-term memories are gradually copied, or **consolidated**, into **long-term memory**, which probably involves permanent structural and physiological changes in brain synapses. Once something has been copied into long-term memory, it can survive lack of attention and even loss of consciousness and may persist for a lifetime.

The Hippocampus and Nearby Cortical Regions Are Critical for Declarative Memory

Key Concepts

The hippocampus is a cortical structure that borders the inferior horn of the lateral ventricle.

The fornix is a prominent output pathway from the hippocampus.

Entorhinal cortex is the principal source of inputs to the hippocampus.

Hippocampal outputs reach entorhinal cortex, the mammillary body, and the septal nuclei.

Bilateral damage to the hippocampus or medial diencephalon impairs declarative memory.

The **hippocampus** is a distinctive area of cerebral cortex folded into the temporal lobe. It is made up of the **dentate gyrus** and the **hippocampus proper**, two interlocking strips of three-layered cortex (unlike the six-layered neocortex described in Chapter 22), together with the **subiculum**, a transition zone between the hippocampus proper and temporal lobe neocortex (Fig. 24-6). The

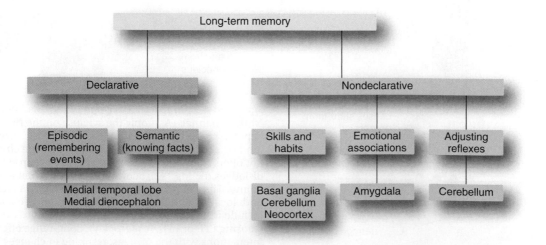

Figure 24-5 Major categories of long-term memory and parts of the CNS prominently involved in each.

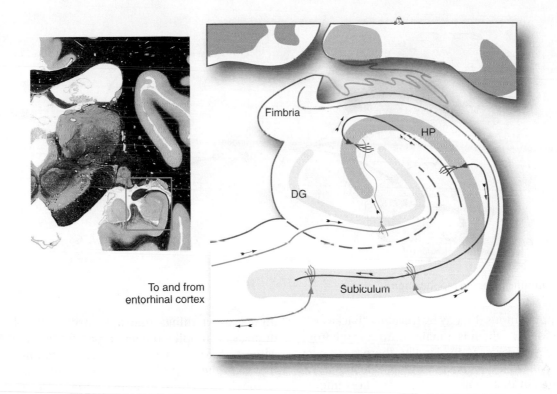

Figure 24-6 Arrangement of cells in a cross section of the hippocampus. Information flows mostly in one direction, arriving from entorhinal cortex and passing through several sequential hippocampal synapses before reaching the subiculum. The fimbria ("fringe") of the hippocampus is the collection of fibers that will leave (or arrive) through the fornix. *DG*, Dentate gyrus; *HP*, hippocampus proper.

anterior part of the **parahippocampal gyrus (entorhinal cortex)** is the major interface between the hippocampus and vast areas of association cortex (see Figs. 24-7 and 24-8), allowing the hippocampus to somehow serve as a key link underlying declarative memory. Bilateral damage to the hippocampus and neighboring areas of cortex, or to the diencephalic areas they are interconnected with, causes **anterograde amnesia**, in which new memories

for facts and events cannot be formed. The **retrograde amnesia** following such damage is not as severe, indicating that long-term memories mostly live outside the hippocampus.

Inputs to entorhinal cortex, and from there to the hippocampus, come from widespread unimodal, multimodal, and limbic areas (Fig. 24-7). In addition, modulatory cholinergic inputs from the septal nuclei

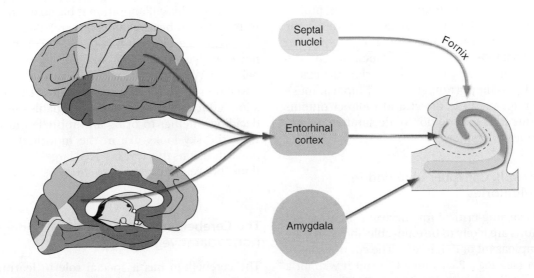

Figure 24-7 Inputs to the hippocampus.

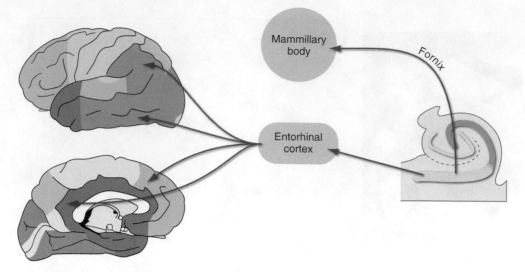

Figure 24-8   Outputs from the hippocampus.

reach the hippocampus directly by traveling "backward" through the **fornix**, which is a major output route from the hippocampus (Fig. 24-8). Finally, there are direct projections from the amygdala to the hippocampus. As discussed later in this chapter, the amygdala is important for marking the emotional significance of situations and events; this connection affects the probability that something will be recorded as a declarative memory, depending on our emotional reaction to it.

The hippocampus then projects back, by way of entorhinal cortex, to widespread unimodal, multimodal, and limbic areas (Fig. 24-8). Hippocampal outputs also reach limbic cortex indirectly, by way of projections to the mammillary bodies through the fornix. The fornix curves around with the lateral ventricle; it separates from the hippocampus near the splenium of the corpus callosum, travels forward along the inferior edge of the septum pellucidum, turns downward in front of the interventricular foramen, and enters the hypothalamus (THB6 Figure 24-17, p. 623). The mammillary bodies project to the **anterior nucleus** of the thalamus through the **mammillothalamic tract**, and this link forms part of a hippocampal loop known as the **Papez circuit** (hippocampus → mammillary body → anterior nucleus → cingulate and parahippocampal gyri → hippocampus). The relative roles of these direct and indirect outputs to limbic cortex in the formation of declarative memories are still not understood.

The Amygdala Is Centrally Involved in Emotional Memories

One form of learning critical for survival is figuring out which situations are likely to be enjoyable and which are likely to be unpleasant or dangerous. The connections of the amygdala (see Figs. 23-7 and 23-8) suit it well for a role in such emotional learning. The amygdala receives inputs about things that are intrinsically pleasant or unpleasant (a full stomach, a painful jab) and is hardwired to have such events cause autonomic reactions (through the hypothalamus) and conscious feelings (through projections to limbic cortex). Information from the thalamus and unimodal sensory areas reaches the same neurons in the amygdala; pairing an otherwise neutral stimulus (e.g., the sight of chocolate or a scorpion) with pleasant or unpleasant outcomes causes activation of NMDA receptors, LTP, and an emotional response to subsequent experience with the previously neutral stimuli.

The Basal Ganglia Are Important for Some Forms of Nondeclarative Memory

Both the basal ganglia and cerebellum collaborate with motor areas of cerebral cortex as we learn to move more rapidly and accurately, as in learning to play a musical instrument; this collaboration is based on the long loops from cortex → basal ganglia or cerebellum → thalamus → cortex (see Figs. 19-2 and 20-7). The basal ganglia, however, have a broader role in learning patterns of behavior. We routinely make decisions about how to act based on subconsciously accumulated experiences that allow "educated guesses" about probable outcomes (e.g., deciding whether to bring an umbrella on the basis of what the sky looks like in the morning). Learning to make decisions this way is based largely on interconnections between the caudate nucleus and association cortex (see Fig. 19-4).

The Cerebellum Is Important for Some Forms of Nondeclarative Memory

The cerebellum has a special role in learning how to adjust movements to fit changing circumstances. This ranges from adjusting the gain of reflexes (e.g., the flocculus changes the gain of the vestibulo-ocular reflex to compensate for wearing eyeglasses) to modifying limb movements (THB6 Figure 20-25, p. 518). The widespread interconnections of the lateral cerebellar hemispheres with nonmotor areas of cerebral cortex indicate that they probably have a broader role in learning various mental skills as well (THB6 Figure 24-24, p. 630).

The powerful excitatory synapses made by climbing fibers on Purkinje cells give the inferior olivary nucleus a particularly important role in cerebellar learning functions.

PNS Repair Is More Effective Than CNS Repair

Once the developmental periods of neuronal death and pruning of connections are finished, the surviving neurons change their patterns of gene expression and concentrate on function and maintenance, rather than growth. This limits the degree of repair after damage, especially in the CNS.

If a neuron in the PNS or CNS is killed by disease or injury, it is generally not replaced (although stem cells, as described a little later, offer some hope for this in the future). If an axon is transected, the part separated from the cell body degenerates (**Wallerian degeneration**, Fig. 24-9). Trophic interactions of the neuron are disrupted, and there may be **anterograde** changes in cells it used to synapse on and **retrograde** changes in neurons that synapse on it. Depending on the neuron's success in regrowing an axon, all of these changes may be reversed or the neuron (or even its synaptic partners) may die.

Peripheral Nerve Fibers Can Regrow After Injury

Following transection of an axon in the PNS, Schwann cells proliferate and secrete trophic factors. In response, the affected neuron ramps up its protein-synthesis machinery and starts to grow a new axon. In the process, even though RNA synthesis increases, Nissl bodies spread out and the cell seems to lose much of its basophilia (**chromatolysis**—"loss of color"). If the regrowing axon successfully reaches its former target, anterograde (e.g., muscle atrophy) and retrograde changes are reversed, and function is restored.

CNS Glial Cells Impede Repair after Injury

The story after transection of an axon in the CNS is different, for two main reasons. First, astrocytes and oligo-

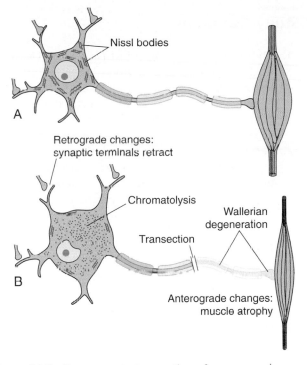

Figure 24-9 Responses to transection of an axon, using a lower motor neuron as an example.

dendrocytes do not secrete trophic factors in response, so the affected neuron is unable to switch on growth-related genes. Second, astrocytes and oligodendrocytes actually interfere with regrowth. Both increase their production of growth-*inhibiting* factors that normally help stabilize connections in adult nervous systems. Astrocytes hypertrophy and wall off the injured area, forming a glial scar that blocks the progress of any regrowing axons. As a result of all this, there is usually a limited chromatolytic response and the axon fails to regrow.

Limited Numbers of New Neurons Are Added to the CNS throughout Life

The conventional wisdom for a long time was that humans are born with all the neurons they will ever have. Recent evidence, however, indicates that there are latent **stem cells**—cells with the potential to produce new neurons—near the walls of all the ventricles, and that there are two locations where new neurons are produced throughout life. Stem cells in the dentate gyrus produce new dentate neurons that may participate in the formation of declarative memories. Stem cells in the wall of the anterior horn of the lateral ventricle produce new inhibitory interneurons that migrate to the olfactory bulb. Coaxing latent or active stem cells to differentiate in controlled ways may make it possible some day to replace lost neurons.

Study Questions

1. There are more lower motor neurons (LMNs) in the L5 spinal cord segment than in T5 because during development
   a. more LMNs are born in L5 than in T5.
   b. more LMNs die in T5 than in L5.
   c. some of the LMNs born in T5 migrate to L5.

2. People tend to have particularly vivid memories of the details surrounding major events in their lives, such as marriages and the birth of children. A major neural connection responsible for the prominence of these memories is that from the ___ to the ___.
   a. amygdala, hippocampus
   b. basal ganglia, hippocampus
   c. basal ganglia, thalamus
   d. cerebellum, amygdala
   e. hypothalamus, hippocampus

3. The term *critical period* refers to a period during which neurons
   a. acquire a permanent identity (e.g., as a cerebral cortical neuron) by brief exposure to critical growth factors.
   b. compete with each other for synaptic sites, resulting in relatively permanent patterns of connections.
   c. migrate from the walls of the neural tube to their final destinations in places like specific layers of the cerebral cortex.
   d. proliferate and have a critical need for growth factors.

4. The majority of fibers in the fornix system connect the ___ to the ___.
   a. amygdala, hypothalamus
   b. amygdala, septal nuclei
   c. cingulate gyrus, parahippocampal gyrus
   d. hippocampus, hypothalamus

5. Following transection of an axon in the adult CNS
   a. the part of the axon distal to the transection regenerates a connection with the parent cell body.
   b. Schwann cells in the vicinity of the transection proliferate and form a scar that blocks regeneration.
   c. oligodendrocytes in the vicinity of the transection secrete substances that actively inhibit regeneration.
   d. the part of the axon distal to the transection degenerates, leaving behind a path through which the proximal part of the axon regrows.

6. Damage to the _____ would be most likely to produce a nondeclarative memory impairment.
   a. anterior nucleus of the thalamus
   b. cerebellum
   c. entorhinal cortex
   d. fornix
   e. hippocampus
   f. mammillary bodies

7. Opening the channel of an NMDA receptor requires simultaneous ___ and ___.
   a. binding of acetylcholine, binding of Mg^{2+}
   b. binding of acetylcholine, depolarization of the surrounding membrane
   c. binding of acetylcholine, hyperpolarization of the surrounding membrane
   d. binding of glutamate, binding of Mg^{2+}
   e. binding of glutamate, depolarization of the surrounding membrane
   f. binding of glutamate, hyperpolarization of the surrounding membrane

For questions 8-10, indicate which of the following CNS components is likely to play the greatest role in that type of learning.
   a. amygdala
   b. basal ganglia
   c. cerebellum
   d. hippocampus

8. Learning to choose the most effective route for driving to school, depending on the weather and the time of day.

9. Keeping track of the meaning of new words and phrases as they come into common usage.

10. Adjusting the force of contraction of the lateral rectus during saccades, in response to minor connective tissue adhesions in the orbit.

Comprehensive Quiz

The material in this study guide, as well as the study questions that go with the material, has thus far been parceled out into (I hope) easy-to-digest chunks. This parceling out, however, is only meant to be a stepwise approach to reaching a broader understanding of the overall organization of the central nervous system. This chapter is a series of questions designed to cover all the material in the book. Some of them are simple review questions referring to individual chapters, whereas others require the integration of material from several chapters. Some have more than one correct answer.

1. Sensory information arriving from one side of the body or head typically reaches the cerebral cortex of the contralateral side. The axons that cross the midline to accomplish this are the axons of

   a. primary sensory neurons.
   b. second-order or higher-order neurons in the sensory pathway.
   c. thalamic neurons.
   d. Could be any of the above, depending on the sensory pathway.

2. Arachnoid villi are

   a. the sites at which cerebrospinal fluid is secreted.
   b. the sites at which cerebrospinal fluid is filtered out of blood.
   c. the sites at which cerebrospinal fluid is pumped out of subarachnoid space and into the venous circulation.
   d. the sites at which cerebrospinal fluid is pushed passively by hydraulic pressure into the venous system.
   e. small vacation homes for spiders in southern France.*

3. As CSF is being withdrawn during a lumbar puncture, the tip of the needle is located in

   a. epidural space.
   b. subarachnoid space.
   c. subdural space.
   d. subpial space.

4. Medial medullary syndrome (the name says something about the location of the lesion) refers to a condition in which a patient has spasticity and diminished proprioception and tactile sensation on one side of the body, combined with weakness and atrophy of the contralateral side of the tongue. Which way would the tongue deviate when protruded? What structures would have been damaged to account for these findings? Occlusion of which artery or arteries would be most likely to cause such a syndrome?

5. A left-handed 65-year-old butterfly collector complains that he has been having more and more difficulty lately collecting butterflies because he "sees double," which confuses him. Your examination reveals a drooping right eyelid, lateral strabismus of the right eye, and a moderately dilated right pupil. He is completely unable to move his right eye to the left past midposition. You can find absolutely no other neurological disturbances. Following angiography, the radiologist announces that the patient has a large intracranial aneurysm. You immediately say, "Aha! I knew it! It's an aneurysm of the …"

---

*Thanks to Dr. Tom Finger.

6. A 39-year-old handball hustler, in an apoplectic rage over a referee's call, suddenly lost consciousness and fell to the floor. He was rushed to an emergency department and treated for an intracranial hemorrhage. When you examine him several days later, you find weakness of his right arm and leg. Stroking the sole of his right foot causes its big toe to turn up and its others to fan. The patient looks at you with his head turned to the left because he says that in any other position he sees double. When you ask him to look straight ahead, his left eye is deviated medially. When you ask him to look to the right, his right eye moves normally and his left eye moves farther medially. When you ask him to look to the left, his right eye again moves normally and his left eye moves laterally almost, but not quite, to midposition. The sensory examination is normal and there are no other cranial nerve findings. Where is the damage? Which artery, or a branch of which artery, caused it?

7. A 33-year-old, right-handed roller derby skater comes to you complaining of periodic attacks of tinnitus ("ringing" or "buzzing") in her left ear and vertigo (the sensation that she and her surroundings are moving relative to one another, when she is standing or sitting still). She says these attacks have been becoming more frequent over the past year or so and that now, between attacks, she feels as though she can't hear as well with her left ear as she can with her right. Your examination reveals that the auditory threshold is indeed elevated in her left ear, whether you use air conduction or bone conduction. You also notice that touching either cornea with a wisp of cotton causes her right eye to blink briskly and her left eye to blink somewhat sluggishly. Then you notice that she seems to have a somewhat asymmetrical smile: The right side of her face moves more than the left. What is the most likely cause of this patient's problems?

8. A 57-year-old, right-handed topologist, while discussing the various routes out of Klein bottles, suddenly became dizzy and tumbled to the floor. She did not lose consciousness but was mildly confused and complained of a severe headache for several days after the fall. Following hospitalization and partial recovery, some symptoms and signs persisted. The patient was referred to you, an eminent neurologist, for diagnosis and treatment 2 weeks after the episode. Your examination revealed the following:

   a. The patient was alert, oriented, intelligent, and showed no sign of confusion.
   b. She no longer complained of headache.
   c. There was complete loss of pain and temperature sensation on the right side of her body.
   d. Her voice seemed hoarse and somewhat abnormal, and her left vocal cord and left soft palate appeared paralyzed.
   e. There was loss of pain and temperature sensation on the left side of her face.
   f. She complained of often feeling dizzy.
   g. Her left arm and leg were mildly ataxic. For example, if she tried to reach for something with her left hand, the hand would oscillate as it approached the object.
   h. Her history revealed that she had enjoyed generally excellent health but had gradually developed hypertension over the previous few years.

Could a single lesion account for all these findings? What structures were damaged? What was the most likely cause?

9. Are there places in the brainstem where a single reasonably discrete lesion could cause:

   a. bilateral Babinski signs?
   b. bilateral loss of tactile and proprioceptive sensation in the entire body?
   c. bilateral loss of pain and temperature sensation in the entire body?
   d. bilateral signs of cerebellar dysfunction?

10. Arrange the following fibers in order of conduction velocity, with the fastest first: afferents from muscle spindles, afferents from temperature receptors, axons of gamma motor neurons.

    a. gamma, temperature, spindle.
    b. gamma, spindle, temperature.
    c. spindle, gamma, temperature.
    d. temperature, gamma, spindle.
    e. spindle, temperature, gamma.

11. A middle-aged neurologist was walking through City Park late one night wearing a peculiar hat and laughing to himself (as he often did) when he was mistaken for a moose by an overeager bowhunter. The left half of his spinal cord was severed at T12. What neurological problems would you expect him to have a month later?

12. Endolymph

    a. fills the bony labyrinth.
    b. fills a restricted part of the membranous labyrinth.
    c. has a high [K⁺], relative to ordinary extracellular fluid.
    d. none of the above.

13. Deafness of the left ear would be caused by damage to the

    a. left cochlear nuclei.
    b. right cochlear nuclei.
    c. left lateral lemniscus.
    d. right lateral lemniscus.
    e. Either a or c.
    f. Either a or d.

14. The visual field deficits shown below (shaded area = defective) could best be explained by

    a. damage in the center of the optic chiasm.
    b. bilateral damage to the temporal lobes.
    c. bilateral damage to the parietal lobes.
    d. damage to the lower half of each occipital lobe.

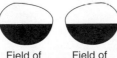

Field of   Field of
left eye   right eye

15. All the following are thalamic relay nuclei *except* the

    a. anterior nucleus.
    b. dorsomedial nucleus (DM).
    c. medial geniculate nucleus.
    d. ventral lateral nucleus (VL).
    e. ventral posteromedial nucleus (VPM).

16. The anterior limb of the internal capsule contains the

    a. auditory radiation.
    b. corticobulbar tract.
    c. corticospinal tract.
    d. efferent fibers from the pulvinar.
    e. thalamic projections to the cingulate gyrus.

Answer questions 17-20 using the following diagram of basal ganglia connections:

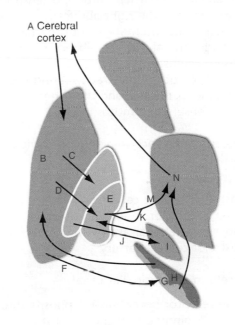

17. Subthalamic fasciculus.

18. VA/VL.

19. Location of neuronal cell bodies that use glutamate as a neurotransmitter.

20. Location of neuronal cell bodies that use GABA as a neurotransmitter.

21. Right hemiballismus would result from damage to the

    a. right subthalamic nucleus.
    b. left subthalamic nucleus.
    c. right globus pallidus.
    d. left globus pallidus.
    e. none of the above.

22. A 37-year-old neuroanatomist and hat designer was involved in a serious collision with a large fish. When you examine him (the neuroanatomist, that is—the fish was unharmed) you notice that when you lightly touch his left cornea, only his left eye blinks; when you touch his right cornea, again only his left eye blinks. Damage in which of the following locations would best account for these findings?

    a. the right oculomotor nucleus, sparing the trigeminal and facial motor and sensory nuclei.
    b. the vicinity of the right abducens nucleus, affecting the internal genu of the facial nerve.
    c. the right spinal trigeminal tract, sparing all other systems.
    d. the left corticobulbar tract, sparing the oculomotor nucleus and the trigeminal and facial sensory and motor nuclei.

23. The caudal pons receives some of its blood supply from the

    a. vertebral artery.
    b. posterior inferior cerebellar artery.
    c. anterior inferior cerebellar artery.
    d. superior cerebellar artery.
    e. posterior cerebral artery.

24. Hair cells in a semicircular canal

    a. have receptor potentials in opposite directions at the beginning and end of a rotation.
    b. continue responding throughout a rotation.
    c. are stimulated best by linear acceleration.
    d. have stereocilia that are bathed in perilymph.

25. Increased stretch reflexes in left lower extremity extensors would result from damage to the

    a. left cerebellar hemisphere.
    b. dopaminergic neurons of the right substantia nigra.
    c. right frontal lobe (areas 4 and 6).
    d. either b or c.
    e. any of the above.

26. Climbing fibers in the left half of the cerebellum originate in the

    a. left pontine nuclei.
    b. right pontine nuclei.
    c. left inferior olivary nucleus.
    d. right inferior olivary nucleus.
    e. none of the above.

27. Most efferents from the putamen project to the

    a. subthalamic nucleus.
    b. caudate nucleus.
    c. VA/VL nuclei of the thalamus.
    d. globus pallidus.
    e. amygdala.

28. The thalamic nucleus most closely associated with parietal-temporal-occipital association cortex is

    a. VPL/VPM.
    b. the dorsomedial nucleus.
    c. the pulvinar.
    d. the anterior nucleus.
    e. the centromedian nucleus.

29. The embryonic diencephalon gives rise to the

    a. putamen.
    b. hypothalamus.
    c. insula.
    d. superior colliculus.
    e. amygdala.

30. Normally present real spaces within the cranium include

    a. subarachnoid space.
    b. subdural space.
    c. epidural space.
    d. a and b.
    e. none of the above.

31. Noncommunicating hydrocephalus would be caused by obstruction of

    a. all three apertures of the fourth ventricle.
    b. one interventricular foramen.
    c. the cerebral aqueduct.
    d. any of the above.
    e. none of the above.

32. A lipid-insoluble dye injected into a lateral ventricle would do all of the following *except*

a. cross the ependymal lining of the ventricle and diffuse between CNS neurons.
b. move through the ventricular system, out into subarachnoid space, and across arachnoid villi, finally entering venous blood.
c. diffuse across the epithelial lining of the choroid plexus and enter choroidal capillaries.
d. stop at tight junctions between the endothelial cells of cerebral capillaries.
e. stop at tight junctions between arachnoid cells.

33. A rapidly aging handball hustler, distracted and upset over missing an easy shot during a match with a medical student, ran into a wall at high speed and was unconscious for several minutes. It was later found that he had suffered anoxic damage to the medial part of both temporal lobes. Which of the following do you think was his biggest problem when he went back to playing handball?

a. He couldn't remember the rules.
b. He had forgotten all his trick shots and couldn't relearn them.
c. He couldn't remember from one day to the next who had won the last game.
d. He had become deaf and couldn't hear the referee's calls.

34. The dorsal motor nucleus of the vagus sends its axons to

a. parasympathetic ganglia.
b. striated muscle of the pharynx.
c. the nucleus of the solitary tract.
d. taste buds in the palate and epiglottis.

35. A 37-year-old goldfish taster comes to your office with a medially deviated right eye, weakness of the entire right side of his face, and inability to move either eye past midposition when he tries to look to the right. A single lesion site that would account for these findings is

a. left frontal cortex, including primary motor cortex and frontal eye fields.
b. right frontal cortex, including primary motor cortex and frontal eye fields.
c. right lateral brainstem at the pontomedullary junction.
d. right medial brainstem in the caudal pons.

36. In both spasticity and parkinsonian rigidity, which of the following is seen in the extensors of the lower extremity?

a. decreased strength
b. increased stretch reflexes
c. increased tone
d. all of the above
e. none of these is seen in both conditions

Use the following list of possible answers for questions 37-40:

a. hippocampus
b. amygdala
c. both
d. neither

37. Is actually an area of cerebral cortex.

38. Receives inputs primarily from entorhinal cortex.

39. Projects to the thalamic dorsomedial nucleus.

40. Has a long output bundle that curves around with the lateral ventricle.

41. Voltage-gated Na^+ channels are found in greatest abundance in which part(s) of a typical neuron?

42. Multiple sclerosis causes focal areas of loss of myelin in the CNS. This demyelinating process involves local loss of or damage to which cell type?

For questions 43-45, choose the most likely site of damage for each case description.

a. left frontal lobe.
b. left parietal lobe.
c. left temporal lobe.
d. right frontal lobe.
e. right parietal lobe.
f. right temporal lobe.

43. A patient who speaks fluently but makes many content errors and has difficulty comprehending both written and spoken language.

44. A patient who ignores one half of his body, failing to dress it and even denying that that side is part of his body.

45. A patient who comprehends the literal meaning of language but who has difficulty distinguishing the emotional intonation in the speech of others.

46. Degeneration of neurons in which part of the brain would cause the most pronounced loss of dopamine in the frontal lobes?

47. Neurons of the _____ have widely branching noradrenergic axons that reach most parts of the CNS.

For questions 48-50, choose the condition from the following list that would best account for the described changes.

    a. blockage of voltage-gated K^+ channels.
    b. blockage of voltage-gated Na^+ channels.
    c. decreased extracellular K^+ concentration.
    d. decreased extracellular Na^+ concentration.
    e. increased extracellular K^+ concentration.
    f. increased extracellular Na^+ concentration.

48. Change in the voltage at the peak of action potentials from +30 mv to +10 mv.

49. Broadening of action potentials, with elimination of the afterhyperpolarization.

50. Diminished size of IPSPs.

Answers

Chapter 1

1. **b.** Lemniscus, fasciculus, and peduncle all refer to white matter structures, leaving putamen as the logical choice. The putamen is in fact a large nucleus that is part of the basal ganglia.

2. **a.** The lenticular nucleus is a major component of the basal ganglia, located subcortically in each cerebral hemisphere (see Fig. 1-1 and Table 1-1).

3. **c.** The midbrain, pons, and medulla are the three subdivisions of the brainstem (see Fig. 1-1 and Table 1-1).

4. **b.** The thalamus and hypothalamus are the major components of the diencephalon (see Fig. 1-1 and Table 1-1).

5. **a.** The amygdala, a major component of the limbic system, is located beneath the medial surface of the temporal lobe (see Fig. 1-1 and Table 1-1).

6. **e.** See THB6 Figure 1-27 (p. 27) for a summary of cell types; also see THB6 Figure 1-30 (p. 29).

7. **f.** See THB6 Figure 1-27 (p. 27) for a summary of cell types; also see THB6 Figure 1-24 (p. 24).

8. **c.** See THB6 Figure 1-27 (p. 27) for a summary of cell types.

9. **b.** Specialized ependymal cells form a secretory epithelium and produce CSF (see Fig. 5-2).

10. **f.** See THB6 Figure 1-27 (p. 27) for a summary of cell types; also see THB6 Figure 1-26 (p. 26).

11. **e.** Kinesin and dynein move organelles along microtubules during fast transport. See THB6 Figure 1-17 (p. 18).

12. **c.** Although synaptic contacts can occur anyplace on a neuron, dendrites are the principal site. See THB6 Figure 8-3 (p. 179) for a beautiful example.

13. **g.** Nissl bodies are large clumps of rough endoplasmic reticulum. See THB6 Figure 1-10, (p. 11).

14. **b.** Although any part of a neuron can be presynaptic in some places, the most common synapses are from axon terminals onto dendrites.

Chapter 2

1. **b.** Defective closure of the neural tube causes malformation of overlying bones. If the rostral neuropore fails to close, anencephaly can result, as in this case.

2. **a.** Neural crest cells give rise to the PNS, including autonomic ganglion cells (see Fig. 2-2).

3. **e.** The skull and face were normal and the cerebral hemispheres present, indicating proper neural tube closure and differentiation of the telencephalon and diencephalon from the prosencephalon. This malformation most likely occurred later in development. See THB6 Figure 2-22B (p. 51).

4. **b.** See Fig. 2-1.

5. **c.** This is the only PNS element among the listed options. (Even though the axons of motor neurons travel through the periphery, their cell bodies reside in the CNS where they were formed.)

6. **c.** See Fig. 2-5.

7. **a.** See Fig. 2-5.

8. **e.** See Fig. 2-5.

9. **b.** See Fig. 2-5.

10. **a.** See Fig. 2-5.

Chapter 3

1. **c.** Postcentral gyrus.

2. **h.** Continues over onto the medial surface of the hemisphere.

3. **c.** Postcentral gyrus, behind the central sulcus.

4. **e.** Visual cortex is located above and below the calcarine sulcus.

5. **f.** The most medial gyrus of the temporal lobe (actually part of the limbic lobe).

6. **h.** Between the midbrain (**g**) and medulla (**i**). Large basal portion protrudes anteriorly.

7. **d.** Posterior enlargement, containing occipital and some parietal and temporal fibers.

8. **c.** The fornix.

9. **f.** The thalamus.

10. **e.** The hypothalamus.

11. **b.** Cortex buried in the lateral sulcus.

12. **c.** Putamen + globus pallidus.

13. **f.**

14. **c.** The lenticular nucleus.

15. **d.** Cortical layer folded into the limbic lobe.

16. **c.** Primary afferents have their cell bodies in places like peripheral ganglia and terminate in the CNS uncrossed.

17. **b.** Because motor neurons almost always project ipsilaterally, **a** is unlikely. In fact, as explained in Chapter 12, the explanation proposed in **b** is correct.

18. **b.** See Fig. 3-8.

19. **d.** Cerebellar damage does not cause sensory deficits; it causes an ipsilateral movement disorder.

20. **d.** See Fig. 3-10.

Chapter 4

1. **a.** Meningeal arteries reside in the periosteal part of the cranial dura, and tears in these arteries can cause separation of the dura from the cranium. See Fig. 4-4.

2. **b.** The cranial dura is attached to the skull externally and the arachnoid internally, so there is no real epidural or subdural space. The pia mater, on the other hand, is attached to the surface of the CNS, leaving a subarachnoid space between itself and the arachnoid. See Fig. 4-1.

3. **a.** The name "dura" is derived from the Latin word for hard or tough (as in durable), describing this thick, collagenous membrane. The arachnoid and pia are much more delicate. See THB6 Figure 4-2 (p. 81).

4. **a.** The cingulate gyrus, just above the corpus callosum, is adjacent to the falx cerebri. See THB6 Figure 4-19C (p. 96).

5. **b.** Cells in a particular layer of the arachnoid are connected to each other by bands of tight junctions, forming a diffusion barrier. See Figs. 4-1 and 6-5.

6. **c.** Arachnoid villi act like holes in the arachnoid barrier layer, allowing passive movement of CSF into dural venous sinuses (see Fig. 4-2).

7. **c.** The meningeal suspension system is made necessary by the *lack* of rigidity of the CNS.

8. **a.** The spinal dura has no periosteal component, so there is a space between the spinal dura and the periosteum of the vertebrae (see Fig. 4-3).

Chapter 5

1. The right lateral ventricle would expand in this case of noncommunicating hydrocephalus. Remaining parts of the

ventricular system would be OK because they still communicate with subarachnoid space and arachnoid villl.

2. **b.** Conventional CT produces maps of x-ray density, so bone is lightest and air is darkest.

3. **d.** See Fig. 3-6.

4. **d.** The median aperture and the two lateral apertures are openings in the fourth ventricle and are the routes through which the ventricular system communicates with subarachnoid space.

5. **a.** Choroid plexus is found in all four ventricles. However, in each lateral ventricle it grows as a single C-shaped strand extending from the inferior horn through the body and then growing through the interventricular foramen. None grows in the anterior horn of the lateral ventricle. See THB6 Figure 5-7 (p. 105).

6. **c.** Choroid epithelial cells are joined to one another by tight junctions, forming a diffusion barrier.

7. **d.** The choroid epithelium is a layer of ependymal cells specialized as a secretory epithelium. Substances that leak across the endothelial and pial layers of the choroid plexus are then actively transported across the choroid epithelium (see Fig. 5-2).

8. Arachnoid villi are the principal routes through which CSF reaches the venous system, and most are located in the walls of the superior sagittal sinus. Anterior occlusions allow CSF to reach most of the villi, but posterior occlusions effectively block this normal route of CSF circulation.

9. **d.** Gray matter, white matter, and CSF have opposite appearances in T1- and T2-weighted images. Bone and air produce little signal in either image type because of the lack of protons (see Fig. 5-6).

10. **e.** b and c both block normal CSF circulation and cause hydrocephalus; in both cases at least part of the ventricular system is cut off from subarachnoid space. a also blocks CSF flow and causes hydrocephalus, but in this case the entire ventricular system is still in communication with subarachnoid

space; hence, **a** would cause *communicating* hydrocephalus.

Chapter 6

1. **d.** Normal cranial nerves indicate the brainstem was probably not affected, eliminating the vertebral artery. Normal visual fields indicate the occipital lobes were probably not affected, eliminating the posterior cerebral artery. The anterior cerebral artery does not supply cortical areas dealing with the face and arm, leaving the middle cerebral artery as the culprit.

2. **c.** The vertebral and posterior inferior cerebellar arteries contribute to the supply of the medulla, the superior cerebellar and posterior cerebral arteries to the rostral pons and midbrain (see Fig. 6-3).

3. **a.** The anterior cerebral artery and its branches parallel the corpus callosum, supplying the cingulate gyrus and the medial surface of the frontal and parietal lobes (see Fig. 6-2).

4. **a.** split between anterior and middle cerebral.
   b. anterior cerebral.
   c.
   d. some middle cerebral, but mostly posterior cerebral.
   e. mostly posterior cerebral and superior cerebellar.
   f. (also a little from the anterior cerebral.)
   g. (also a little from the anterior cerebral.)
   h. posterior cerebral.

5. There might be no effect in either case because under normal circumstances little blood flows through either artery. If perforating branches of one or both communicating arteries were involved, some deficits due to diencephalic damage might be noted.

6. **c.** See Fig. 6-4.

7. **d.** On its way to the occipital lobe, the posterior cerebral artery supplies medial and inferior parts of the temporal lobe (see Fig. 6-2).

8. **b.** Distal branches of the middle cerebral artery are distributed to the lateral surface of the hemisphere and feed into the system of superficial veins (see Fig. 6-6). The internal cerebral vein is part of the system of deep veins.

9. **c.** See Fig. 6-5. Choroidal capillaries, unlike usual CNS capillaries, are fenestrated; the pia mater is freely permeable at all locations.

10. **a.** Autoregulation keeps the total blood flow to the brain relatively constant. Local metabolic changes result in increased flow to active areas balanced by decreased flow to relatively inactive areas.

Chapter 7

1. **a.** Closing K^+ channels would increase the relative permeability of the membrane to Na^+, so the membrane potential would move closer to V_{Na}.

2. **b.** Closing Na^+ channels would increase the relative permeability of the membrane to K^+, so the membrane potential would move closer to V_K. (In typical neurons this would be a very small hyperpolarization because there's not much Na^+ permeability to begin with and the membrane potential is already close to V_K.)

3. **a.** This would move V_{Na} to a more positive value. Because the membrane potential is a weighted average between V_K and V_{Na}, a small depolarization would result.

4. **b.** This would move V_K to a more negative value. Because the membrane potential is a weighted average between V_K and V_{Na}, hyperpolarization would result.

5. **a.** Lack of pumping would allow the Na^+ and K^+ concentration gradients to dissipate, moving the membrane potential to or toward 0 mv.

6. **a.** A large diameter makes it easier for current to travel down the dendrite, and few open channels make it harder for current to leave; both factors increase the length constant.

7. **b.** Lowered V_{Na}, lowered peak of the action potential.

8. **a.** Prolonged action potential, lack of an afterhyperpolarization.

9. **c.** Prolonged action potential, but an afterhyperpolarization is still present, indicating the opening of K^+ channels.

10. **c.** Both larger diameter and the presence of myelin increase conduction velocity.

Chapter 8

1. **a.** See Table 8-1.

2. **d.** Neuropeptides are synthesized and packaged in the cell body, then shipped down the axon; small-molecule transmitters are synthesized by soluble enzymes in synaptic endings.

3. **a.** Acetylcholine is the major PNS excitatory transmitter, in this case acting at nicotinic receptors.

4. **f.** GABA is the principal CNS inhibitory transmitter.

5. **a.** Acetylcholine is the major PNS excitatory transmitter, here again acting at nicotinic receptors.

6. **e.** Glutamate is the major excitatory transmitter in the CNS, used at something like 90% of CNS synapses.

7. **f.** GABA is the principal CNS inhibitory transmitter.

8. **b.** Degeneration of the pigmented, dopaminergic neurons of the substantia nigra (compact part) causes Parkinson's disease (see Fig. 11-9 and Chapter 19).

9. **e.** Glutamate is the principal CNS excitatory transmitter.

10. **c.** With few exceptions, postsynaptic effects are not mediated by voltage-gated channels. Of the ligand-gated channels listed, only the opening of a Na^+/K^+ channel would cause depolarization.

Chapter 9

1. **d.**

2. **e.** Receptor potentials spread electrotonically, like postsynaptic potentials.

3. **b.** Notice that the receptor responds vigorously while the stimulus is changing but stops responding when the stimulus is constant.

4. **b.** See Fig. 9-5.

5. **b.** Stimulating gamma motor neurons causes contraction of the ends of intrafusal fibers. This in turn stretches the central part of the intrafusal fibers, where the stretch receptor endings are applied, and makes the primary afferents fire faster. See THB6 Figure 9-15 (p. 217).

6. **a, c.**

7. **e.** Kind of a trick question, but most touch receptors are medium diameter and many are thinly myelinated or unmyelinated. See THB6 Table 9-3 (p. 224).

8. **a, c.**

9. **b, d.** (Although some are thinly myelinated, many are unmyelinated.)

10. **b, d.**

11. **c.** The epineurium is continuous with the dura mater and shares its mechanical strength. See THB6 Figure 9-19 (p. 222).

12. **c.** The perineurium is continuous with the arachnoid (see THB6 Figure 9-19, p. 222) and contains a continuation of the arachnoid barrier layer.

Chapter 10

1. The first thing to go would be the fibers crossing in the anterior white commissure to form the spinothalamic tracts of both sides at that level. This would lead to loss of pain and temperature sensation bilaterally in the dermatomes represented by fibers crossing in the damaged segments (dermatomes would correspond to spinal levels 1-2 segments caudal to the actual damage; see THB6 Figure 10-22, p. 248). Subsequent damage is variable but typically involves nearby lower motor neurons, causing weakness and eventually atrophy of muscles innervated by affected segments. See THB6 Figure 10-32 (p. 263) for an actual case.

2. Segments affected can be determined on the basis of the reflexes affected. Then the appropriate dermatomes can be tested for sensory loss. Also, ventral root damage eventually results in muscle atrophy, whereas dorsal root damage does not. Perhaps most simply, the patient will still be able to contract the muscle voluntarily if its afferent innervation is defective, even though reflexes involving the muscle may be hypoactive.

3. Weakness of all extremities suggests bilateral damage to lateral corticospinal tracts. Bilateral deficits of pain and temperature sensation suggest damage to lateral spinothalamic tracts on both sides. Together these findings imply damage to both lateral funiculi. Intact tactile sensation implies intact posterior columns. The anterior spinal artery (see THB6 Figures 10-29 and 10-30, pp. 261 and 262) supplies the entire cord except for the posterior horns and posterior columns, and its occlusion could produce such damage extending over one or several segments. Supply of the lateral corticospinal tract may be partially from the posterior spinal artery, so the degree of weakness is variable from one case to another. This is the classic anterior spinal artery syndrome.

4. **d.** Part of the cervical enlargement.

5. **a.** There are only eight cervical segments.

6. **c.** Preganglionic sympathetics from T1-L3.

7. **b.** See Fig. 10-1.

8. **d.** Spinothalamic tract.

9. **b.** Fasciculus cuneatus, large-diameter primary afferents (including those from muscle spindles) from the upper extremity.

10. **e.** Primary afferents usually don't cross the midline.

11. **c.** Lateral corticospinal tract.

12. **e.** See Fig. 10-3.

13. **c.** a and b are incorrect (see Fig. 10-8), and c describes the general function of sympathetics.

Chapter 11

1. **d.** This one is subtle. The left-sided weakness and Babinski sign are consistent with brainstem

damage on the right. The incoordination implies damage to the cerebellum or its connections. To explain incoordination of the left limbs caused by damage on the right, you need to find a place where, for example, cerebellar outputs have crossed on their way to the thalamus. The rostral midbrain, above the decussation of the superior cerebellar peduncles (see THB6 Figures 11-17 and 20-22, pp. 280 and 514), is such a place.

2. **e.** See Fig. 11-7.

3. **d.** See Fig. 11-6.

4. **a.** See Fig. 11-2.

5. **b.** See Fig. 11-3.

6. **d.** See Fig. 11-6.

For 7-11, see THB6 Figure 11-30 (p. 292).

7. **d** or **f.**

8. **b.** (some contribution from **a** and **e**).

9. **a.** (with contributions from **b**).

10. **c.**

11. **d.**

12. **b.** Degeneration of the pigmented, dopaminergic neurons of the substantia nigra (compact part) causes Parkinson's disease (see Chapter 19).

13. **d.** Raphe nuclei (see Fig. 11-10).

14. **c.** See Fig. 11-8.

15. **a.** See Fig. 11-11.

Chapter 12

1. **f.** Right ptosis and lateral strabismus: right CN III, implying right midbrain damage. Left weakness and Babinski: right cerebral peduncle (midbrain).

2. **a.** Right weakness, Babinski, impaired touch and position sense: left corticospinal tract and medial lemniscus. Left tongue weakness: left hypoglossal nerve or nucleus (medulla), or

possibly right corticobulbar tract. Because the long tract signs indicate left-sided damage, left hypoglossal damage is most likely. This is the medial medullary syndrome (see Fig. 12-11).

3. **e.** This time the limb and tongue weakness is all on the left, suggesting corticospinal/corticobulbar damage. The weak right lateral rectus (CN VI) places the damage in the right side of the pons.

4. **a.** Lateral medullary syndrome (see Fig. 12-11).

5. **b.** These are in the glossopharyngeal nerve.

6. **c.** Primary afferents almost always end ipsilaterally and do not reach the thalamus. The trigeminal main sensory nucleus takes care of touch.

7. Yes, because the main sensory nucleus is lateral to the motor nucleus, corresponding to their derivations from alar and basal plates.

8. **d.** See Fig. 12-6.

9. **d.** See Fig. 12-9.

10. **b.** See Fig. 12-2.

11. **b.** The trigeminal nerve (as it leaves the brainstem) contains somatic sensory fibers and motor axons to the masseter and other muscles.

12. **d.** No hypoglossal fibers, no olfactory information, the solitary tract terminates in the nucleus of the solitary tract.

13. Assuming only one of the four nerves is damaged, then when you stroke the left cornea:
    If both eyes blink, the left trigeminal and both facial nerves must be OK;
    if neither eye blinks, the left trigeminal nerve must be damaged;
    if only the left eye blinks, the right facial nerve must be damaged;
    if only the right eye blinks, the left facial nerve must be damaged.

14. Three examples: corneal abrasion from foreign objects due to loss of the blink reflex; chewing damage to the inside of the cheek due to loss of sensation; drooling and loss of food from one

side of the mouth, also due to loss of sensation. All these effects would be on the side ipsilateral to the treatment.

Chapter 13

1. **c.** Basic taste sensations are intact (solitary tracts OK). Sharp "smells"—common chemical sense—intact (lingual nerves OK).

2. **d.** No hypoglossal fibers, no olfactory information, the solitary tract terminates in the nucleus of the solitary tract.

3. **b.** See Fig. 13-5.

4. **b.** See Fig. 13-1.

5. **c.** Taste receptor cells have no axons and use both G protein-coupled mechanisms and other mechanisms. See THB6 Figure 13-5 (p. 328).

Chapter 14

1. **a.** The left stapedius does not contract under any circumstances, indicating left facial nerve damage. Sound in the left ear can make the right stapedius contract, indicating that left CN VIII is OK. See Fig. 14-6.

2. **a.** This is a selective problem with air conduction in the right ear. Bone conduction in both ears is apparently normal, ruling out **b** and **c**. Neither **d** nor **e** would cause a pronounced unilateral problem.

3. **c.** Perilymph *surrounds* the membranous labyrinth; the vestibule is part of the bony labyrinth and contains the saccule and utricle.

4. **d.** See Figs. 14-1 and 14-2.

5. **a.** The mechanical advantage of the ossicles is slight.

6. **a.** Endolymph has a high [K⁺] and low [Na⁺], and synapses could not work in this environment. The helicotrema connects two perilymph-filled compartments.

7. **d.** The basilar membrane is wider and floppier toward the apex of the cochlea, and so resonates at lower frequencies.

8. **a.** See Fig. 14-4 (or THB6 Figure 14-11, p. 354).

9. **c.** Cochlear primary afferents end uncrossed in the cochlear nuclei. At all levels rostral to this, information from both ears is compared. See Fig. 14-5.

10. **c.** See THB6 Figure 14-18 (p. 359).

11. **a.** The semicircular ducts respond best to changes in angular velocity, the saccule to tilts starting from a head-sideways position.

12. **b.**

13. **c.** Vestibular nystagmus does not persist during maintained rotation. See Fig. 14-8 (or THB6 Figure 14-33, p. 373).

Chapter 16

1. **e.** Somatosensory relay nucleus for the body.

2. **d.** Association nucleus for prefrontal cortex.

3. **f.** Relay nucleus for vision (the pulvinar also projects to parts of the occipital lobe).

4. **e.** Somatosensory relay nucleus for the body.

5. **a.** Limbic relay nucleus.

6. **c.** Auditory relay nucleus.

7. **b.** Motor relay nucleus.

8. **a.** On their way to the cingulate gyrus.

9. **b.** See THB6 Figures 18-12 and 18-13 (p. 467).

10. **c, d.** See THB6 Figure 17-28 (p. 442).

11. **b.** The posterior limb is adjacent to VPL.

Chapter 17

1. **d.** Left nasal hemianopia: only one eye affected, so it must be due to a lesion in front of the optic chiasm or on the side of the optic chiasm.

2. **f.** Left optic tract damage → right homonymous hemianopia. (Could also be **l**.)

3. **a.** Left optic nerve damage → blind left eye.

4. **h.** Fibers representing upper visual field quadrants go through the sublenticular part of the internal capsule and Meyer's loop.

5. **b.** Damage to crossing fibers in the optic chiasm (from nasal halves of the retinas) → bitemporal hemianopia.

6. **l.** Left visual cortex damage → right homonymous hemianopia, often with macular sparing.

7. **b.** See Fig. 17-2.

8. **b.** The optic nerve leaves the back of the eye a little medial to the fovea. Because the optics reverse everything, the blind spot is a little lateral to the fovea in the visual field. See THB6 Figure 17-32 (p. 445).

9. **a.** The fovea is a region of tightly packed cones.

10. **c.** Fibers on their way to the lower bank of the calcarine sulcus, representing upper quadrants of the visual field, pass through the sublenticular part of the internal capsule.

11. **b.** The left half of each retina (i.e., the right visual field) is represented in the left occipital lobe, and the fovea projects to the posterior part of the occipital lobe. See THB6 Figure 17-29 (p. 443).

12. **b.** Asymmetrical pupils usually mean damage to the motor nerves supplying the iris. A large pupil implies an unopposed dilator, caused by oculomotor damage; lack of a light response confirms this. (Another possibility is damage to the iris itself.)

13. **b.** Cones are not forced to take care of only color vision. For example, you are using your foveal cones to read this black-and-white print.

14. **b.** See Figs. 17-8 and 17-9.

15. **b.** See Fig. 17-3.

Chapter 18

1. **c.** Among the listed structures, only damage to the internal capsule would cause weakness (see Fig. 18-4).

2. **b.** The thalamus only projects to other forebrain structures, primarily the cerebral cortex.

3. **e.** See THB6 Figure 18-10 (p. 464).

4. **a.** See Fig. 18-5.

5. **e.** a and b are characteristics of lower motor neuron damage, c and d of upper motor neuron damage.

6. **d.** Corticospinal fibers cross in the pyramidal decussation, so c would have ipsilateral effects.

7. **d.** Motor neurons for muscles of the larynx, pharynx, and upper face receive bilateral corticobulbar innervation. See Fig. 18-7.

8. **f.** See THB6 Figure 18-6 (p. 460).

Chapter 19

1. **e.** Flailing movements of both limbs on one side typify hemiballismus. Basal ganglia disorders are seen contralateral to a lesion.

2. **a.** "Strio-" indicates that the fibers originate in the caudate, putamen, or ventral striatum; "-nigral" indicates that they end in the substantia nigra.

3. **d.** The caudate nucleus receives most of its cortical inputs from association areas, the putamen from somatosensory and motor areas, and the ventral striatum from limbic structures (see Fig. 19-4).

4. **a.** See Fig. 19-2.

5. **c.** Rigidity is not characterized by weakness or increased reflexes, and spasticity is not characterized by tremor at rest. However, rigidity includes increased tone of most or all muscles and spasticity includes increased tone in upper extremity flexors. So both conditions have increased biceps tone in common.

6. **d.** See Fig. 19-1.

7. **m.** In the principal circuit linking basal ganglia and cerebral cortex, pallidothalamic fibers travel through the lenticular fasciculus (**l**) and the ansa lenticularis (**k**), which join with cerebellar efferents to form the thalamic fasciculus.

8. **i.** Inputs from GPe, outputs to GPi.

9. **h.** Dopaminergic outputs from SNc to the striatum (and other parts of the basal ganglia).

10. **b, e,** and **g.** Outputs from the striatum, globus pallidus, and SNr are all GABAergic.

11. **i.** The subthalamic nucleus is the principal source of excitatory (glutamate) projections *within* the basal ganglia.

Chapter 20

1. **a.** See Fig. 20-4.

2. **c.** Mossy and climbing fibers are cerebellar afferents. Only a few Purkinje axons leave the cerebellum; most project to the deep nuclei, which in turn provide the cerebellar output (see Fig. 20-3).

3. **a.** See Fig. 20-5.

4. **d.** See Fig. 20-5.

5. **a.** See Fig. 20-1.

6. **a.** The vermis and medial hemisphere receive most of the spinal afferents to the cerebellum; the vermis is concerned with the trunk, the medial hemisphere with the extremities.

7. **c.** This information must cross the midline someplace in order to keep both the left side of the cerebellum and the right cerebral hemisphere related to the left side of the body. The superior cerebellar peduncles are efferent from the cerebellum, and the thalamus does not project to the pons.

8. **a.** Climbing fibers come from the contralateral inferior olivary nucleus and make up the bulk of the inferior cerebellar peduncle (see Fig. 20-2A).

9. **c.** Except for efferents to the vestibular nuclei and reticular formation (which go through the inferior peduncle), almost all cerebellar efferents travel through the superior cerebellar peduncle (see Fig. 20-2A).

10. **a.** Through the juxtarestiform body, part of the inferior cerebellar peduncle.

11. Because olivocerebellar fibers (i.e., climbing fibers) are crossed, spino-olivary fibers would also need to cross the midline in order to keep one side of the cerebellum related to the same side of the body.

Chapter 21

1. **c.** Voluntary eye movements (saccades) to the contralateral side are triggered from the frontal eye field (see Fig. 21-4). Tracking movements involve more posterior cortical areas. Damage to the abducens nucleus would affect both types of movement. (Another possible site of damage to account for this problem would be the right PPRF.)

2. **c.** Convergence does not require medial rectus-lateral rectus coordination.

3. **e.** The superior oblique reaches across the top of the eye and pulls toward the nose, intorting the eye. See THB6 Figure 21-7B (p. 528).

4. **a.** Abduction depends mostly on the lateral rectus (CN VI), and the oculomotor nerve makes a relatively small contribution by way of the inferior oblique.

5. **b.** The flocculus plays a critical role in VOR suppression and adaptation.

Chapter 22

1. **d.**

2. **d.**

3. **i.** Primary visual cortex.

4. **c** (also **k**). Agranular cortex contains many large pyramidal cells with long axons. Primary motor cortex is the premier example.

5. **h.** Parietal lobe, especially the superior part.

6. **m.** The cingulate gyrus, which, together with the parahippocampal gyrus, makes up nearly all of the limbic lobe.

7. **l.** Anterior to primary motor cortex, on the medial surface of the hemisphere.

8. **l.** Premotor and supplementary motor cortex.

9. **f.** Wernicke's area.

10. **b.** Damage to the nondominant inferior frontal gyrus causes problems generating prosody; damage to the nondominant superior temporal gyrus causes problems comprehending it.

11. **e.** Much of the basic machinery for both kinds of sleep is in the brainstem. The EEG of REM sleep is comparable to the EEG when awake and alert, whereas the EEG during slow-wave sleep is large and slow. **b** and **c** are characteristics of REM sleep.

Chapter 23

1. **c.** See THB6 Figure 23-3 (p. 583).

2. **c.** See Fig. 23-2.

3. **d.** See Fig. 22-6.

4. **d.** See Fig. 23-5.

5. **b.** The stria terminalis, a relatively small pathway in humans, travels in the wall of the lateral ventricle carrying fibers to and from the amygdala. See THB6 Figure 23-20 (p. 600).

6. **d.** 4 in Fig. 22-5.

7. **g.** During the storage phase sympathetics inhibit the detrusor, parasympathetics are relatively silent, and the pontine micturition center is turned off (see Fig. 23-6A).

8. **e.** See Fig. 23-7.

9. **b.** See Fig. 23-8.

10. **b.** The amygdala forms memories of the emotional significance of objects and events, and the hypothalamus triggers the autonomic reactions. This is discussed a little more in Chapter 24.

Chapter 24

1. **b.** Neurons are overproduced during development, and excess neurons die off, throughout the nervous system.

2. **a.** Although the hippocampus is centrally involved in the formation of declarative memories, inputs from the amygdala affect the probability that a declarative memory of some event will be formed at all.

3. **b.** a, c, and d all happen before connections are refined during critical periods.

4. **d.** See Fig. 24-8.

5. **c.**

6. **b.** All the other options are related to the hippocampus and declarative memory.

7. **e.** See Fig. 24-4.

8. **b.** This is the kind of nondeclarative memory, based on slowly learned probabilities, that the basal ganglia are involved in. See THB6 Figure 24-23 (p. 629).

9. **d.** Knowing the meaning of words is a form of declarative memory.

10. **c.** The cerebellum excels at adjusting movements to fit circumstances.

Appendix 1: Comprehensive Quiz

1. **b.** Neither primary afferents nor thalamocortical axons typically cross the midline (see Fig. 3-8).

2. **d.** See Fig. 4-2.

3. **b.** The lumbar cistern is a CSF-filled subarachnoid space. See Fig. 4-3.

4. Tongue deviates toward the weak side; damage to the corticospinal tract, medial lemniscus, and hypoglossal nerve on one side (see Fig. 12-11); anterior spinal or (more likely) vertebral artery.

5. All these findings could be explained by damage to the right third nerve (selective damage to one oculomotor nucleus is very rare). As THB6 Figure 6-3 (p. 125) shows, an aneurysm at any of several locations near the bifurcation of the basilar artery could be responsible. In fact, the site of origin of the posterior communicating artery is most likely.

6. Weakness of the right arm and leg, with Babinski sign, implies damage to the right lateral corticospinal tract high in the spinal cord, or the left corticospinal tract somewhere rostral to the spinal cord. The eye movement disorder indicates damage to the left abducens nerve and places the lesion on the left side of the caudal pons. See THB6 Figure 15-6 (p. 384). Damage here, involving a perforating branch of the basilar artery, would account for the findings. (AICA supplies an area dorsolateral to this.)

7. The elevated auditory threshold on the left side indicates damage to the left CN VIII or the left cochlear nuclei (but not a more rostral location in the auditory system). Nerve damage seems more likely because there are no signs of cerebellar damage, even though the inferior cerebellar peduncle is adjacent to the cochlear nuclei. CN VIII damage would also explain the vertigo. The asymmetrical smile and the sluggish blink reflex indicate damage to the left facial nerve or nucleus. Cranial nerves VII and VIII are close together (see Fig. 12-1) in the cerebellopontine angle, and the findings can be most easily accounted for by a tumor in this region (e.g., a vestibular schwannoma).

8. This is a variation on the classic lateral medullary (Wallenberg's) syndrome (see Fig. 12-11). The left vertebral or posterior inferior cerebellar artery is the most likely culprit. **c** = damage to left spinothalamic tract; **d** = damage to left nucleus ambiguus; **e** = damage to left spinal trigeminal tract; **f** = damage to left vestibular nuclei; **g** = damage to left inferior cerebellar peduncle.

9. **a,** Medullary pyramids or pyramidal decussation. **b,** Crossing internal arcuate fibers in the medulla, or both medial lemnisci where they are adjacent to the midline in the rostral medulla. **c,** No; the spinothalamic tracts are never near the midline in the brainstem. **d,** Decussation of the superior cerebellar peduncles in the caudal midbrain; or conceivably, in the rostral medulla affecting crossing fibers from both inferior olivary nuclei; or crossing fibers in the basal pons on their way to the middle cerebellar peduncles.

10. **c.** Muscle spindle afferents are large and heavily myelinated, gamma axons medium sized, and fibers from temperature receptors small and thinly myelinated or unmyelinated (see Fig. 9-7).

11. Ipsilateral spastic weakness below T12 (corticospinal tract), ipsilateral tactile and proprioceptive deficit below T12 (fasciculus gracilis), and contralateral pain and temperature loss beginning a little below T12 (spinothalamic tract). This is called the Brown-Séquard syndrome. See THB6 Figure 10-31 (p. 262).

12. **c.** Endolymph fills the entire membranous labyrinth, so **a** and **b** are incorrect, and endolymph does in fact have the peculiar composition described.

13. **a.** Afferents from the left cochlea end in the left cochlear nuclei; thereafter, the information is distributed bilaterally (see Fig. 14-5).

14. **c.** **a** would cause bitemporal hemianopia; **b** and **d** would cause *superior* homonymous hemianopia (see Fig. 17-5).

15. **b.** The dorsomedial nucleus is the association nucleus for prefrontal cortex. See THB6 Figure 16-18 (p. 404).

16. **e.** efferents from the anterior nucleus (see Table 16-1). All the others are in the posterior limb (**b, c, d**) or in the retrolenticular (**d**) or sublenticular (**a, d**) part.

17. **j.** Fibers traveling in both directions across the internal capsule to interconnect the subthalamic nucleus (**i**) and the globus pallidus. See THB6 Figure 19-16 (p. 486).

18. **n.** VA/VL is the motor relay part of the thalamus.

19. **a, i,** and **n.** Outputs from the cortex, subthalamic nucleus, and thalamus all use glutamate.

20. **b, e,** and **g.** Outputs from the striatum, globus pallidus, and SNr are all GABAergic.

21. **b.** Damage to the subthalamic nucleus is associated with hemiballismus. See THB6 Figure 19-21C (p. 490). Basal ganglia connections are mostly contained within a cerebral hemisphere, so damage affects the contralateral side.

22. **b.** The right orbicularis oculi, controlled by the right facial nerve, is not working (see Fig. 12-8). (Additional deficits would be expected if the MLF or abducens nucleus were damaged.)

23. **c.** **a** and **b** supply the medulla, **d** the rostral pons/caudal midbrain, and **e** the midbrain and thalamus (see Fig. 11-12).

24. **a.** Endolymph keeps moving for a little while at the end of rotation, causing a reversal in the relative direction of flow (see Fig. 14-8).

25. **c.** Cerebellar damage often causes decreased reflexes; Parkinson's disease typically is not accompanied by reflex changes.

26. **d.** Climbing fibers originate from the inferior olivary nucleus, cross the midline, and enter the cerebellum through the inferior cerebellar peduncle (see Fig. 20-2A).

27. **d.** The major basal ganglia circuit is striatum → globus pallidus → thalamus → cerebral cortex → striatum (see Fig. 19-5).

28. **c.** See THB6 Figure 16-18 (p. 404).

29. **b.** The putamen, insula, and amygdala are telencephalic derivatives. See Fig. 2-5.

30. **a.** Subdural and epidural spaces can become actual spaces as a result of certain hemorrhages (see Fig. 4-4) , but subarachnoid space is the only one normally present.

31. **d.** In all of these situations, part (or all) of the ventricular system is no longer in communication with subarachnoid space.

32. **c.** The choroid epithelium is part of the CNS barrier system (see Fig. 6-5), so solutes don't diffuse across it.

33. **c.** Medial temporal damage does not wipe out all old memories or affect skills; auditory cortex is located more laterally, in the transverse temporal gyri.

34. **a.** The major parasympathetic nucleus of the brainstem (see Fig. 12-2).

35. **d.** Weakness of the entire right half of the face indicates damage to the right facial nerve or nucleus in the caudal pons. The eye movement syndrome, called a "one and a half" (see THB6 Figure 12-10, p. 305), confirms this.

36. **c.** Neither strength nor reflexes are affected in parkinsonian rigidity. Tone is increased everywhere in rigidity, however, and is disproportionately increased in upper extremity flexors and lower extremity extensors in upper motor neuron disease.

37. **a.** Three-layered cortex, but still cortex.

38. **a.** See Fig. 24-7.

39. **b.** And from there to orbital and anterior limbic cortex. See Fig. 23-8.

40. **c.** See THB6 Figures 23-20 and 24-17 (pp. 600 and 623).

41. In the trigger zone for initiation of action potentials (usually assumed to be the axon initial segment), and along the axon (unmyelinated axon) or at nodes of Ranvier (myelinated axon).

42. Oligodendrocytes, which form myelin sheaths in the CNS.

43. **c.** Wernicke's aphasia (usually involves damage more widespread than just Wernicke's area).

44. **e or f.** Contralateral neglect, traditionally said to be most common following right parietal damage (although right temporal lobe damage may be at least as important).

45. **f.** The prosody equivalent of Wernicke's aphasia.

46. The ventral tegmental area, which projects to frontal cortex and limbic structures (see Fig. 11-9).

47. Locus ceruleus (see Fig. 11-8).

48. **d.** Decreased Na^+ concentration gradient moves V_{Na} to a lower voltage.

49. **a.** Voltage-gated K^+ channels are a major component of the repolarization mechanism, and the increased K^+ permeability they cause accounts for the afterhyperpolarization.

50. **e.** Typical IPSPs are caused by increased K^+ or Cl^- permeability. Decreasing the K^+ concentration gradient causes changes in K^+ permeability to have less effect.

Blank Drawings

These are laid out in about the same order in which they appeared in the text of *The Human Brain,* 6th ed. You may find them useful for self-quizzing or review.

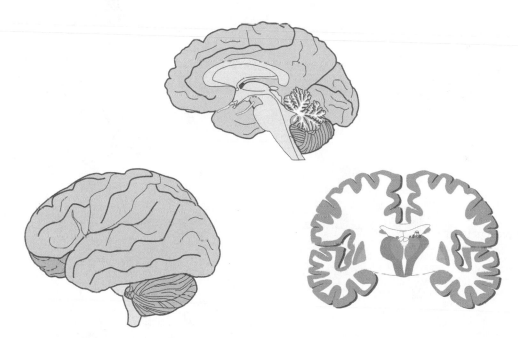

Figure A3-1 Major parts of the brain.

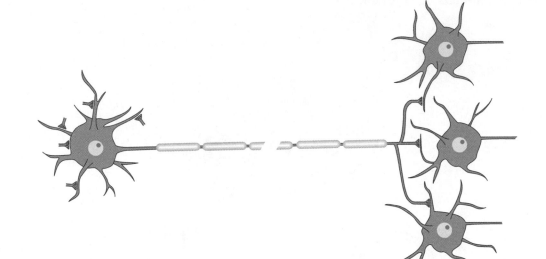

Figure A3-2   Typical neuron.

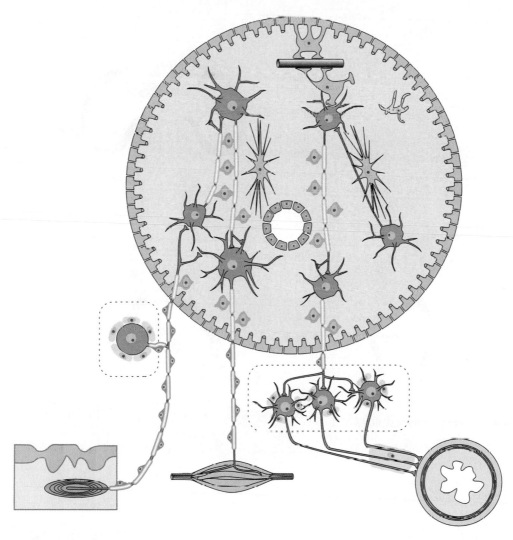

Figure A3-3 Cell types in the PNS and CNS.

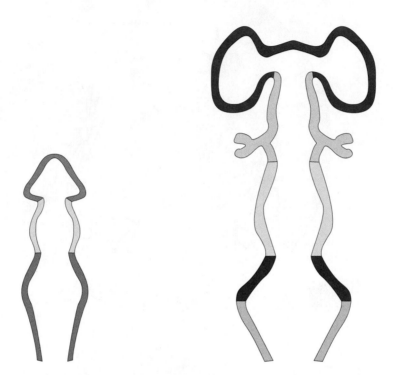

Figure A3-4   Primary and secondary vesicles of the neural tube.

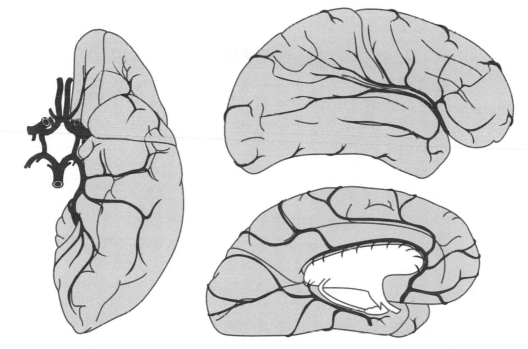

Figure A3-5   Cerebral arterial supply. *(Modified from Mettler FA: Neuroanatomy, ed 2. St. Louis, Mosby, 1948.)*

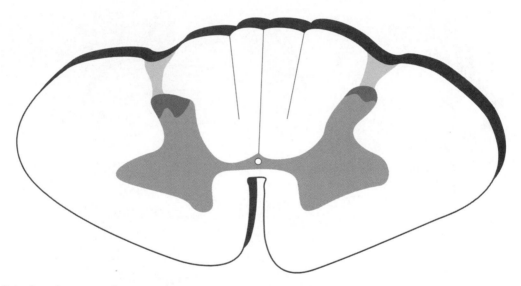

Figure A3-6 Spinal cord cross section.

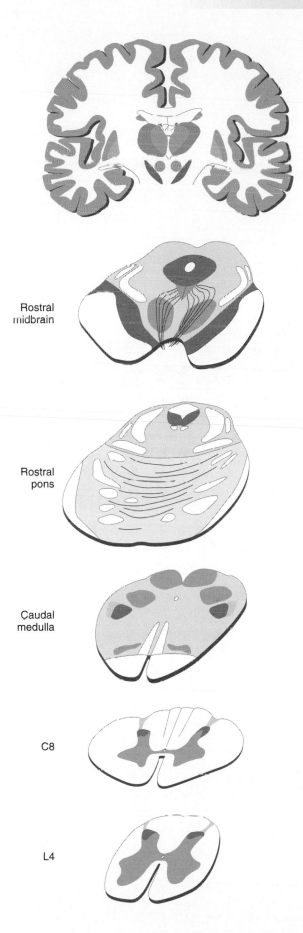

Rostral
midbrain

Rostral
pons

Caudal
medulla

C8

L4

Figure A3-7 Long tracts.

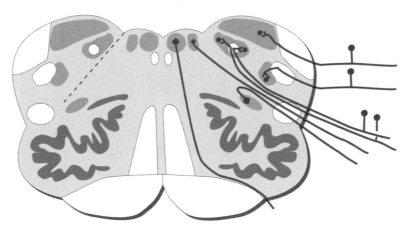

Figure A3-8   Cranial nerve nuclei.

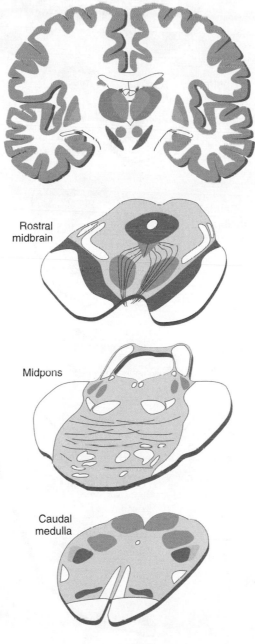

Rostral
midbrain

Midpons

Caudal
medulla

Figure A3-9 Trigeminal connections.

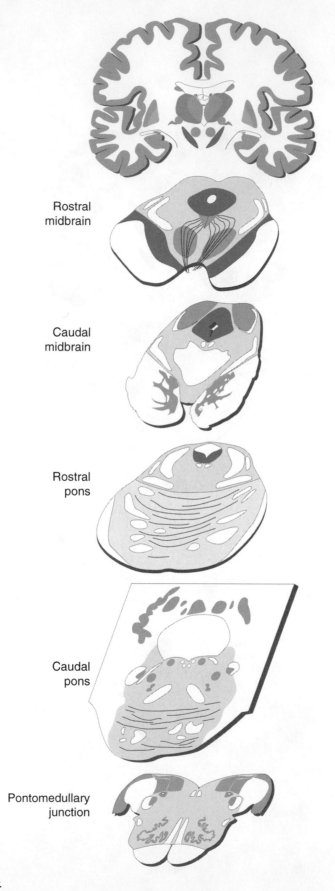

Rostral
midbrain

Caudal
midbrain

Rostral
pons

Caudal
pons

Pontomedullary
junction

Figure A3-10   Auditory pathway.

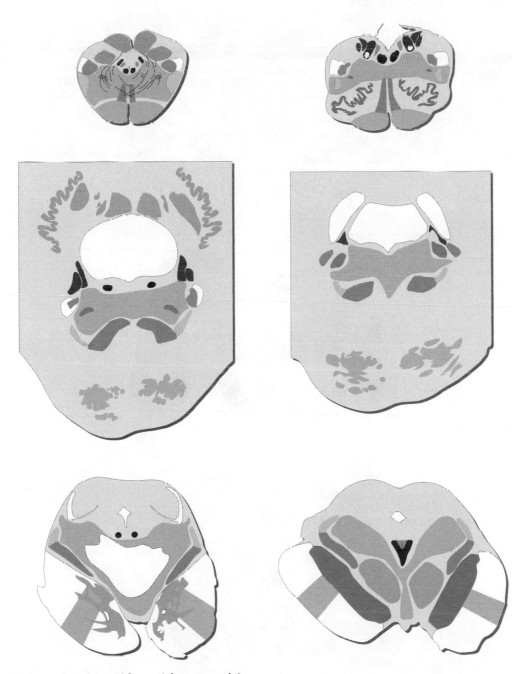

Figure A3-11 Brainstem sections with cranial nerve nuclei.

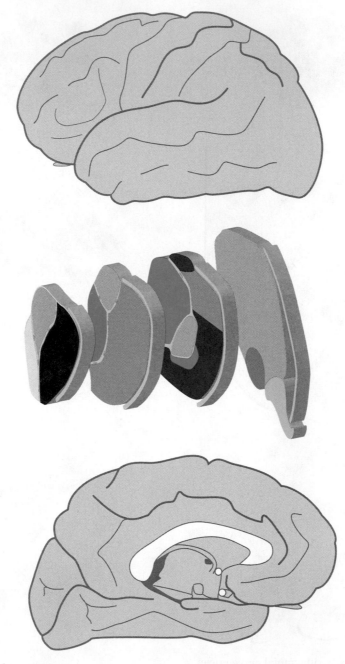

Figure A3-12   Thalamocortical connections.

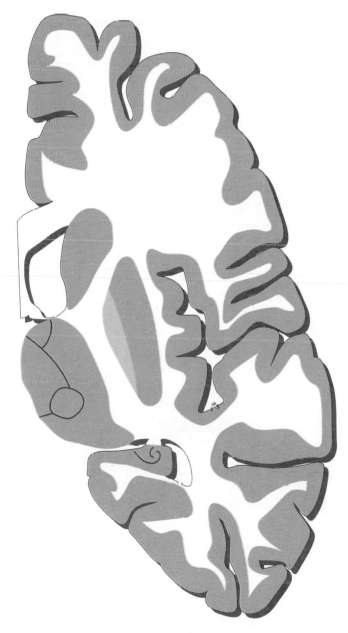

Figure A3-13   Thalamus and internal capsule.

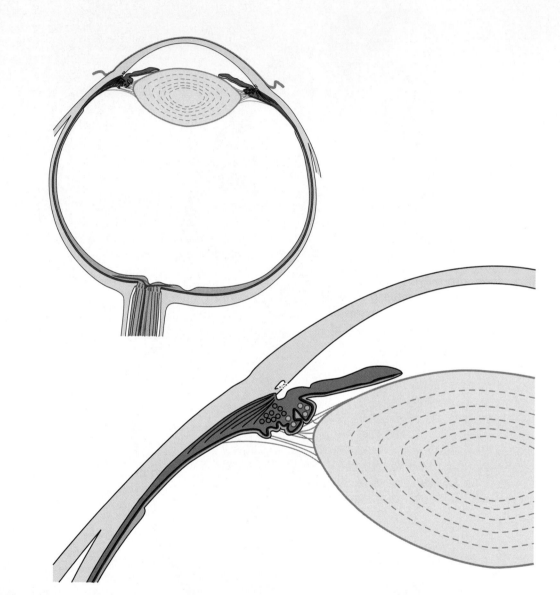

Figure A3-14   Eye.

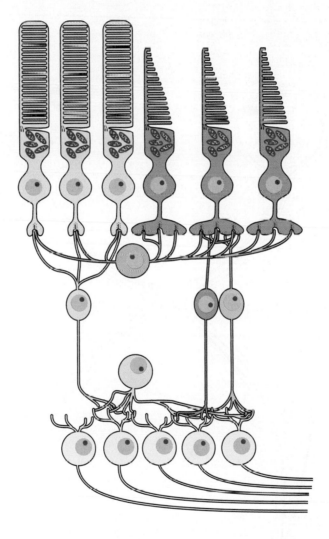

Figure A3-15   Retina.

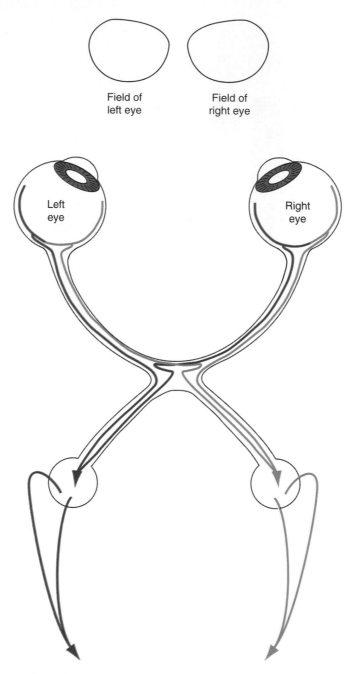

Figure A3-16 Visual pathway and visual fields.

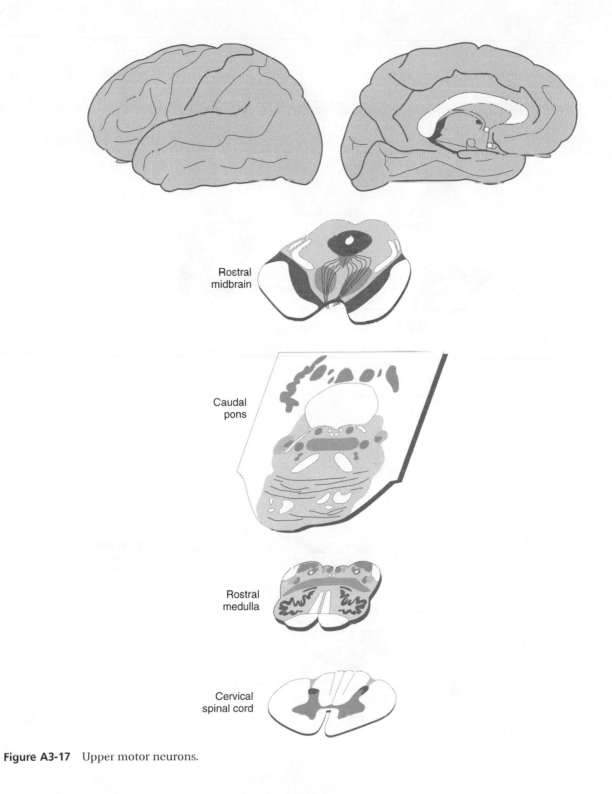

Rostral
midbrain

Caudal
pons

Rostral
medulla

Cervical
spinal cord

Figure A3-17   Upper motor neurons.

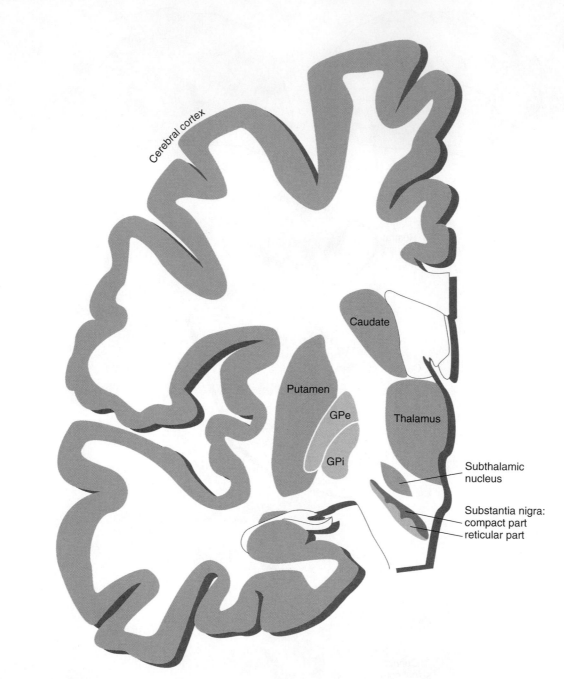

Figure A3-18 Basal ganglia.

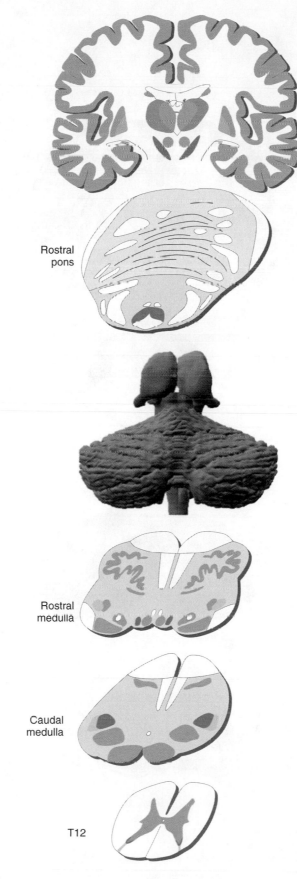

Rostral
pons

Rostral
medulla

Caudal
medulla

T12

Figure A3-19 Cerebellar inputs.

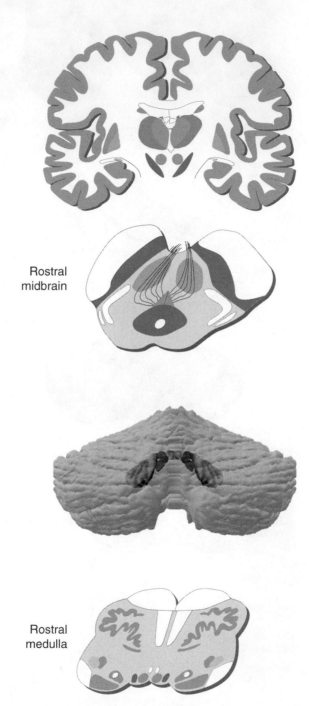

Rostral
midbrain

Rostral
medulla

Figure A3-20 Cerebellar outputs.

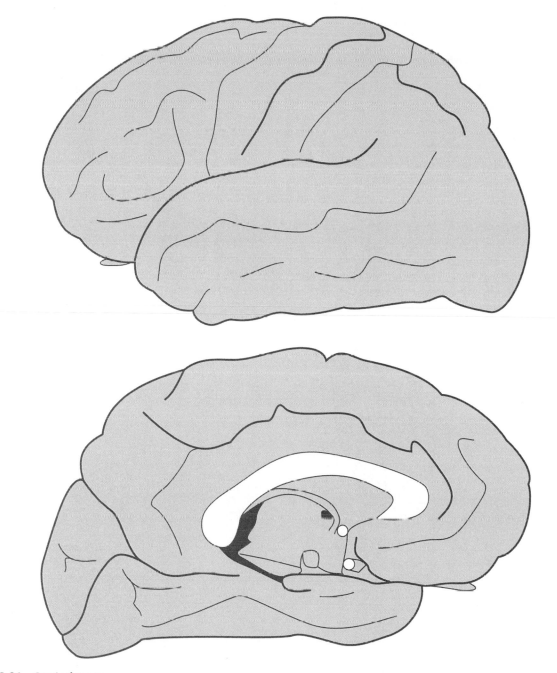

Figure A3-21 Cortical areas.

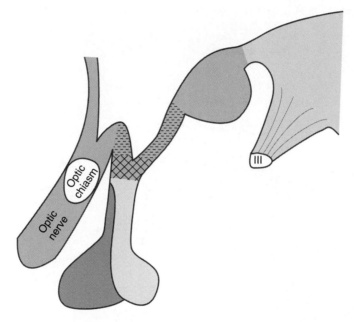

Figure A3-22 Hypothalamus.

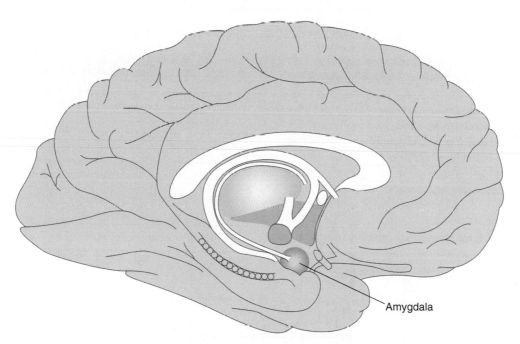

Amygdala

Figure A3-23   Connections of the amygdala. *(Modified from Warwick R, Williams PL: Gray's Anatomy, Br ed 35. Philadelphia, WB Saunders, 1973.)*

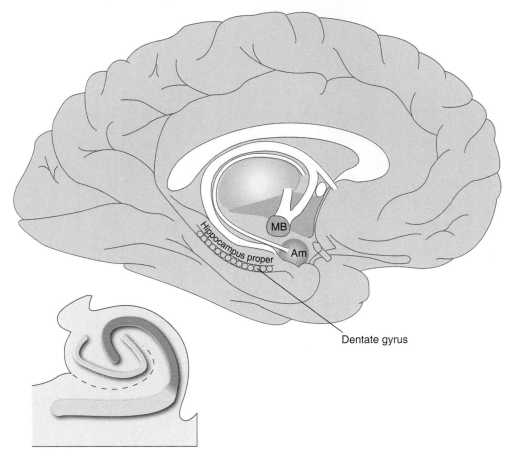

Figure A3-24 Connections of the hippocampus. *(Upper part modified from Warwick R, Williams PL: Gray's Anatomy, Br ed 35. Philadelphia, WB Saunders, 1973.)*

Index